Pritikin Diet
For Seniors

The Complete Guide To Weight Loss And Improved Health For Seniors

Samantha Bax

Pritikin Diet For Seniors
Samantha Bax

Prose Books
Prose Books LLC
Merrimack, NH 03054 USA
email: info@prosebooks.us

Table of Contents

Chapter 1: Introduction

Introduction to the Pritikin Diet

In today's paced and convenience-driven society, seniors face increasing challenges in maintaining health and managing their weight. As we age, our bodies undergo changes that make weight management and overall well-being vital for a fulfilling life.

The Pritikin Diet offers a proven solution for seniors who want to improve their health, shed pounds, and boost their overall vitality. This chapter serves as an introduction to the Pritikin Diet, highlighting the significance of weight management for seniors and showcasing the benefits of this dietary approach.

The Significance of Weight Management for Seniors

Weight management plays a role in ensuring seniors' well-being and overall health. As we get older, our metabolism naturally slows down, with a decline in muscle mass and physical activity levels. These factors, lifestyles, and poor dietary choices make seniors more vulnerable to weight gain and related health issues. Obesity or excess weight can lead to problems like heart disease, diabetes, high blood pressure, joint pain, and even certain types of cancer. Additionally, carrying weight can worsen existing health conditions while reducing the quality of life for seniors.

Maintaining a weight goes beyond how we look; seniors must achieve and sustain a healthy body mass index (BMI) to prevent or manage chronic diseases and enhance their lifespan. By embracing the Pritikin Diet, seniors can take charge of their weight. Significantly lower the risk of developing these health conditions, enabling them to lead a fulfilling and active life well into their golden years.

Advantages of the Pritikin Diet for Seniors

The Pritikin Diet is a regarded and evidence-based approach that has proven effective for individuals of all ages, including seniors. This diet focuses on foods with plant-based options that are dense in nutrients but low in calories while minimizing the consumption of highly processed and calorie-dense choices. By following the principles of the Pritikin Diet, seniors can enjoy benefits, including:

Weight Management: The Pritikin Diet is designed to facilitate sustainable weight loss. By prioritizing foods and low-calorie alternatives, seniors can achieve a body weight while reducing stress on their joints and enhancing overall mobility.

Heart Health: Seniors are particularly susceptible to heart disease, which is a leading cause of mortality in this age group. The Pritikin Diet is well known for its ability to lower cholesterol, decrease blood pressure, and prevent heart disease. By following this approach, seniors can safeguard their heart health. Potentially reverse existing heart conditions.

Managing Diabetes: Type 2 diabetes is an ailment among seniors often associated with food choices and excess weight. The Pritikin Diet emphasizes index foods and eliminates refined sugars to promote healthy blood sugar control. Seniors who adhere to this diet can better manage their diabetes. Reduce the risk of developing it.

Boosting Nutrient Intake: As we age, our bodies have requirements. The Pritikin Diet ensures that seniors receive vitamins, minerals, and antioxidants for optimal health. By including a variety of fruits, vegetables, whole grains, and lean proteins in their meals, seniors can enhance function, support brain health, and reduce the risk of age-related diseases.

Increased Energy and Vitality: Seniors who embrace the Pritikin Diet often report energy levels, improved sleep quality, and an overall boost in vitality. This nutrient-rich diet provides seniors with the fuel to engage in physical activity while promoting mental well-being for a better quality of life.

As we begin our exploration of the Pritikin Diet, it's crucial to recognize how important weight management is for individuals and the many advantages this dietary method can bring. By emphasizing foods supporting weight loss and prioritizing heart health and diabetes control, the Pritikin Diet offers seniors a solution for achieving and maintaining optimal well-being.

In the sections, we will delve deeper into the principles and guidelines of the Pritikin Diet, providing seniors with the knowledge and resources they need to embrace this transformative approach to healthy living.

Chapter 2: Understanding Weight Management in Seniors

As people grow older, managing weight becomes increasingly crucial for maintaining health and well-being. Seniors face challenges in terms of weight gain and loss, which can have an impact on their quality of life. In this chapter, we will explore the factors that affect weight gain and loss in seniors, including changes in metabolism, fluctuations in hormones, and common obstacles to losing weight. Understanding these factors is essential for developing strategies to help seniors maintain weight and enhance their overall well-being.

Factors Influencing Weight Gain and Loss in Seniors

Changes in Metabolism as We Age: One of the factors that influence weight management among seniors is the decline in metabolic rate that occurs as we get older. Metabolism refers to the processes through which our bodies convert food into energy. With age, our metabolism slows down, resulting in a decrease in the number of calories burned while at rest. This reduction in metabolic rate makes it easier to gain weight and more challenging to shed pounds. Therefore, seniors need to adjust their caloric intake and engage in activity to counteract this decline.

Impact of Hormonal Changes on Weight: Hormonal changes also play a role when it comes to managing weight among seniors. As men and women age, there is a decrease in hormone production, such as testosterone and estrogen. These fluctuations in hormones can cause an increase in body fat and a reduction in muscle mass, leading to weight gain. Furthermore, imbalances in hormones can impact appetite and the body's ability to regulate blood sugar levels, making it more challenging to manage weight. By understanding how hormonal changes affect seniors, both seniors themselves and healthcare professionals can develop targeted strategies to effectively manage weight.

Challenges Seniors Face in Losing Weight: Seniors often encounter obstacles when trying to lose weight.

These obstacles include:

a. Chronic Health Conditions: Many seniors deal with health conditions like arthritis, cardiovascular diseases, or diabetes. These conditions can limit their activity levels, making it more difficult for them to manage their weight. Additionally, certain medications used for treating these conditions may have effects that contribute to weight gain.

b. Reduced Mobility: Age-related factors like decreasing muscle strength and joint stiffness can restrict seniors' mobility. This decrease in activity can lead to weight gain. Hinder their efforts to lose weight. Exploring low-impact exercises and customized physical activity programs can help seniors overcome this obstacle.

c.. Social Factors: The emotional and social aspects play a role in how seniors eat and take care of their well-being. Feelings like loneliness, depression, or stress can influence their eating habits. Sometimes, they resort to comfort foods, which can lead to gaining weight. It is important to acknowledge and address these social factors when it comes to managing weight.

Moreover, seniors often face challenges that require attention. These challenges include reduced appetite, difficulties with chewing or swallowing, and limited access to foods. These factors can result in nutrient intake, leading to weight loss or malnutrition. To overcome these challenges, it is crucial to provide seniors with guidance and ensure they have access to nutrient-rich foods.

Furthermore, as people age, they may experience changes in their sense of taste and smell. This can result in decreased enjoyment of food for seniors, causing them to consume calories overall. However, it can also make them prefer high-calorie foods. Understanding these changes enables tailoring recommendations that make mealtimes more enjoyable for seniors.

Maintaining weight is vital for the health and well-being of seniors.

It is essential to comprehend the factors that contribute to weight gain or loss among individuals—factors such as changes in metabolism, hormonal fluctuations, and common obstacles faced when trying to lose weight. This understanding helps develop strategies for managing weight.

By taking these factors into consideration and implementing strategies, healthcare providers, caregivers, and older adults can collaborate to support seniors in maintaining weight and improving their overall quality of life.

Chapter 3: The Principles of the Pritikin Diet

Understanding the Basics of the Pritikin Diet

In our quest for health and well-being, it is vital to grasp the principles that form the foundation of the Pritikin Diet. Developed by scientist and nutritionist Dr. Nathan Pritikin, this dietary approach has transformed our perspective on nutrition and its impact on our well-being. By adopting a diet that's low in fat and high in fiber, prioritizing foods, and acknowledging the importance of regular exercise for weight management, the Pritikin Diet offers a holistic and effective strategy to enhance both our physical and mental health.

Emphasizing a Low Fat, High Fiber Approach

The principle of the Pritikin Diet revolves around consuming a diet that's low in fat but abundant in fiber. This principle stems from research highlighting the adverse effects of excessive fat intake on our health. By reducing our consumption of saturated and trans fats, we can significantly reduce our risk of developing conditions such as heart disease, diabetes, and certain types of cancers.

Instead of relying on fats for energy, the Pritikin Diet encourages individuals to incorporate substantial amounts of dietary fiber into their meals. Fiber plays a role in digestion as it supports bowel movements while also assisting in regulating blood sugar levels. Furthermore, including fiber foods helps promote feelings of fullness or satiety, which can reduce overeating tendencies.

You can find plenty of it in fruits, vegetables, whole grains, and legumes.

When we include these fiber foods in our meals, we can enhance our overall well-being while still enjoying a satisfying and nourishing diet.

Emphasis on Whole Foods

Another crucial aspect of the Pritikin Diet is its focus on food. Processed and refined foods often contain additives that lack the nutrients our bodies require for optimal performance. On the other hand, whole foods provide us with a wide range of essential vitamins, minerals, and phytonutrients that are vital for our health.

Whole foods like fruits and vegetables, whole grains, lean proteins, and plant-based fats offer benefits to our health. They contribute to strengthening our system, boosting energy levels, improving digestion, and supporting brain function. By prioritizing these choices in our diet, we can improve our well-being while also savoring the delightful variety of flavors and textures they provide.

The Significance of Regular Exercise in Managing Weight

While following a diet is fundamental to leading a lifestyle, the Pritikin Diet acknowledges that weight management involves multiple aspects. In addition to adjusting, incorporating exercise is crucial for achieving and maintaining a healthy weight.

Regular physical exercise has benefits not only for weight loss but also for our overall well-being. It helps boost our metabolism, making it easier to burn calories efficiently when combined with a diet. Moreover, exercise contributes to building muscle mass, resulting in better body composition and increased strength. Additionally, engaging in activities has an impact on reducing stress levels, improving mood, and enhancing mental clarity.

Incorporating exercise into our routine doesn't necessarily mean spending hours at the gym. Enjoyable activities like walking, cycling, swimming, or dancing can be equally effective in promoting weight management and overall fitness. The Pritikin Diet emphasizes finding a balance between workouts, strength training exercises, and flexibility routines to create a rounded and sustainable fitness plan.

By understanding the principles of the Pritikin Diet, we empower ourselves to make choices about our health and well-being.

Its focus on high-fiber foods, along with the importance of regular exercise, lays the foundation for adopting a healthier lifestyle centered around whole foods. By embracing these principles, we can set ourselves on a path toward attaining peak health and vitality.

Chapter 4: Getting Started with the Pritikin Diet

Before starting any diet plan, it's important to evaluate your eating habits. This step allows you to identify areas where you can make improvements and understand the adjustments needed to follow the Pritikin Diet.

To begin, keep a food journal for at least one week. Write down everything you eat and drink, including portion sizes and the time of day. This record will give you insights into your eating patterns. Help you recognize any unhealthy habits or behaviors that might be impacting your weight management goals.

As you review your food journal, pay attention to the types of foods you consume. Are you eating a balanced diet with plenty of fruits, vegetables, whole grains, and lean proteins?. Is your diet primarily focused on processed foods, sugary snacks, and unhealthy fats? Understanding your eating habits will guide you in making changes that support a healthier lifestyle.

Once you have evaluated your eating habits, it's time to set goals for weight management. Remember that successful and sustainable weight loss is a process that requires patience and dedication.

To achieve weight loss, it is advisable to aim for a steady reduction of 1 2 pounds per week. Rapid weight loss can have effects on your well-being.

Consider seeking guidance from a registered dietitian or healthcare professional who can assist you in setting goals based on your needs and circumstances. They will provide advice on how to reach a weight range while ensuring you receive adequate nutrition and maintain optimal energy levels.

When establishing your weight management goals, it is important to focus not on the number displayed on the scale but on enhancing your overall health. Strive to lower the risk of conditions like heart disease and diabetes by adopting eating habits and making positive lifestyle choices.

Developing a Personalized Meal Plan

For adherence to the Pritikin Diet, it is crucial to create a meal plan that suits your individual preferences and requirements. This meal plan should be balanced, nutrient-rich, and sustainable in the run.

Begin by dividing your plate into portions: allocate half for starchy vegetables, one quarter for whole grains or starchy vegetables, and one quarter for lean proteins. Include amounts of fats, like nuts, seeds, or avocado, in each meal to support satiety and overall well-being.

When planning your meals, prioritize foods that are minimally processed.

To maintain a diet, it's important to incorporate a variety of fruits, vegetables, whole grains, legumes, and lean proteins into your meals. Try to limit your intake of added sugars, unhealthy fats, and processed foods. Opt for high-fiber options as they support digestion and help you stay fuller for periods.

It's also an idea to diversify your meal choices so that you can get a range of essential nutrients. Experiment with cooking techniques, flavors, and textures to make your meals interesting and enjoyable. Use herbs, spices, and natural condiments to enhance the taste without adding calories or sodium.

When it comes to grocery shopping and meal preparation on the Pritikin Diet journey, there are some tips:

Plan: Create a meal plan for the week and make a shopping list with all the necessary ingredients. This will prevent purchases.

Focus on produce: Shop around the perimeter of the store, where you'll find fresh fruits, vegetables, lean meats, and low-fat dairy products. Try to minimize your time in the processed food aisles.

Read labels: Take some time to read ingredient lists and nutrition facts on packaged items. When you're looking for products, try to find ones that have amounts of added sugars, unhealthy fats, and sodium. It's also an idea to choose grain options whenever possible.

- **Opt for produce that's in season:** These items tend to be the most nutritious and flavorful. Buying a variety of fruits and vegetables will keep your meals interesting.

- **Planning:** Take some time each week to pre-portion and batch-cook your meals. This way, you can easily grab an option when you're on the go.

- **Experiment:** Experiment with cooking techniques that don't rely heavily on added fats. Grilling, steaming, baking, or sautéing with oil or using stick pans are great alternatives.

By following these suggestions, you'll make your shopping experience more efficient, save time, and set yourself up for success in sticking to the Pritikin Diet.

This chapter has highlighted the importance of evaluating your eating habits, setting weight management goals, creating a personalized meal plan, and implementing effective strategies for grocery shopping and meal preparation. By incorporating these elements into your journey with the Pritikin Diet, you're building a foundation for long-term success in achieving a lifestyle.

In the chapters, we will explore further the elements of the Pritikin Diet. This will help you gain an understanding and equip you with the resources needed to accomplish your health and well-being objectives.

Chapter 5: Meal Planning and Recipes

As we grow older, our dietary requirements. It has become crucial to be more mindful of our food choices. Having a planned and balanced diet can greatly impact our health and well-being. In this section, we will explore the significance of meal planning for seniors.

We discussed how incorporating the principles of the Pritikin Diet into our meals can bring numerous benefits. Additionally, we will introduce you to some nutritious recipes based on the Pritikin Diet that will be featured in sections, making it a delightful experience to embrace healthy eating.

Understanding how much we eat is vital when it comes to maintaining weight and preventing illnesses. As we age, our metabolism tends to slow down, resulting in reduced calorie requirements. By comprehending portion control, we can ensure that we consume an amount of food that meets our needs without overindulging.

One effective approach for portion control involves using cues as guides. For instance, a serving size of protein should resemble a deck of cards in terms of dimensions, while cooked vegetables or whole grains should be around the size of a tennis ball. It is also important to pay attention to the recommended number of servings for each food group.

The guidelines provided by the USDA's MyPlate offer a framework for managing portion sizes. Highlight the importance of including fruits, vegetables, whole grains, lean proteins, and low-fat dairy in our everyday diet.

Integrating Pritikin Diet Principles into Our Regular Meals

The Pritikin Diet, created by Nathan Pritikin, centers around consuming foods that are rich in nutrients while limiting saturated fats, cholesterol, and sodium. This diet is well known for its impact on heart health, blood pressure reduction, and weight loss. By incorporating the principles of the Pritikin Diet into our meals, we can enjoy the benefits of a lifestyle.

The core principles of the Pritikin Diet involve including a variety of fruits, vegetables, whole grains, and lean proteins in our diet while minimizing processed foods, sugary drinks, and fatty dairy products. This approach encourages us to consume foods that provide essential vitamins, minerals, and antioxidants to support overall well-being.

By giving priority to foods in our meal plans, we can savor an array of flavors and textures while providing our bodies with the necessary nourishment. In sections or chapters in this guidebook or article series, we will explore an assortment of delicious yet nutritious recipes that adhere to the principles of the Pritikin Diet. These recipes will demonstrate how you can easily incorporate these principles into your day-to-day meals.

Now that we understand how important it is for seniors to plan their meals and control portion sizes let us dive into the world of nutritious Pritikin Diet recipes. In the chapters, you'll discover a range of tasty dishes that not only satisfy your taste buds but also provide the necessary nutrients for seniors.

These handpicked recipes are designed to cater to seniors' needs while ensuring they enjoy every bite. From nourishing soups and vibrant salads to fulfilling courses and mouthwatering desserts, these recipes will inspire you to create enjoyable meals.

Each recipe will include a list of ingredients, step-by-step instructions, and nutritional information. This way, you'll have all the information to make choices about what you eat. Following the principles of the Pritikin Diet, we'll explore a world of culinary delights that will boost your well-being and leave you feeling revitalized.

In this chapter, we've discussed how crucial meal planning is for seniors and highlighted the benefits of incorporating Pritikin Diet principles into our meals.

By having a grasp of portion control and prioritizing rich foods in nutrients, we can keep our weight in check, enhance the health of our hearts, and overall improve our well-being. In the following sections, we will introduce you to a variety of mouthwatering and nourishing recipes from the Pritikin Diet that will turn your meals into beneficial moments. Prepare yourself for an adventure filled with nourishment and taste.

Chapter 6: Breakfast Recipes

Welcome to Chapter 6 of "***The Pritikin Diet for Seniors: The Complete Guide to Weight Loss and Improved Health for Seniors***." Breakfast holds importance as it kickstarts your day with a nourishing and fulfilling meal, setting the tone for a vibrant day ahead. In this chapter, we will explore a variety of breakfast recipes tailored to support weight management and enhance overall well-being for seniors.

These recipes not only taste delicious, but they are also carefully designed to provide essential nutrients, keep you satiated, and boost a healthy metabolism. We understand that breakfast should be both nourishing and enjoyable, which is why we have curated a selection of dishes catering to tastes and preferences.

Whether you crave breakfast classics, prefer something wholesome, or seek inventive savory options, this chapter offers something for everyone. You will find recipes incorporating grains, lean proteins, and an abundance of fruits and vegetables to help you maintain a healthy body weight while relishing the flavors in each bite.

As we delve into the recipes, within this chapter, you will discover that embracing eating can be a gratifying journey.

Alright, let us begin this journey together and kickstart your day the Pritikin way with some breakfast recipes that not only fuel your body but also help you manage your weight and promote a long and healthy life.

Chapter 1: Pritikin Breakfast Delights

1. Quinoa and Mixed Berry Bowl with Citrus Zest

2. Flaxseed and Oat Bran Muffins with Fresh Berries

3. Spinach and Mushroom Breakfast Scramble (no oil)

4. Chilled Melon Soup with Fresh Mint

5. Whole Grain Toast with Smashed Avocado and Cherry Tomatoes

6. Barley and Vegetable Hash with Fresh Herbs

7. Steel-cut oats with Cinnamon, Apple, and Walnuts

8. Broccoli and Red Pepper Egg White Omelette

9. Fresh Fruit Salad with a Splash of Orange Juice

10. Rye Pancakes Topped with Stewed Berries (no added sugars)

11. Zucchini and Corn Breakfast Burritos (whole grain tortillas)

12. Banana and Blueberry Smoothie with Chia Seeds (no added sugars)

13. Lentil and Kale Morning Stew

14. Pineapple and Mango Overnight Oats with Almond Slivers

These recipes are more in line with the principles of the Pritikin Diet, focusing on whole foods, low-fat content, and minimal sugars.

Recipe 1: Quinoa and Mixed Berry Bowl with Citrus Zest

Prep Time: 10 minutes - Cooking Time: 20 minutes - Number of Servings: 4

Ingredients:

- 1 cup uncooked quinoa rinsed and drained.
- 2 cups water
- 2 cups mixed berries (blueberries, strawberries, raspberries, blackberries)
- Zest of 1 lemon
- Zest of 1 orange
- 2 tsp pure vanilla extract
- 2 tbsp honey or maple syrup (optional for added sweetness)
- A pinch of salt
- Fresh mint leaves for garnish (optional)

Instructions:

1. In a medium-sized saucepan, combine quinoa, water, and a pinch of salt. Bring to a boil.

2. Reduce heat to low, cover, and simmer until quinoa is tender and water is absorbed, about 15 minutes.

3. Remove from heat and let it stand for 5 minutes. Then, fluff with a fork.

4. While the quinoa is still warm, stir in the vanilla extract and honey or maple syrup if using.

5. Divide quinoa among bowls. Top with mixed berries.

6. Sprinkle the citrus zest over the berries.

7. Garnish with fresh mint leaves if desired.

8. Serve warm or at room temperature.

Nutritional Values (per serving):

- Calories: 200

- Protein: 6g

- Carbohydrates: 39g

- Dietary Fiber: 5g

Cooking Tip: For a creamier texture, you can stir in a dollop of low-fat Greek yogurt or almond milk before adding the berries.

Recipe 2: Flaxseed and Oat Bran Muffins with Fresh Berries

Prep Time: 15 minutes - Cooking Time: 20-25 minutes - Number of Servings: 12 muffins

Ingredients:
- 1 cup oat bran
- 1/2 cup ground flaxseed
- 1 cup whole wheat flour
- 2 tsp baking powder
- 1/2 tsp baking soda
- 1/4 tsp salt
- 2 large eggs, beaten.
- 1/4 cup honey or maple syrup
- 1 tsp pure vanilla extract
- 1 cup unsweetened applesauce
- 1/2 cup almond milk (or any milk of choice)
- 1 cup mixed fresh berries (like blueberries, raspberries, chopped strawberries)

Instructions:
1. Preheat the oven to 375°F (190°C). Line a muffin tin with paper liners or lightly grease.
2. In a large mixing bowl, whisk together oat bran, ground flaxseed, whole wheat flour, baking powder, baking soda, and salt.
3. In another bowl, combine the beaten eggs, honey or maple syrup, vanilla extract, applesauce, and almond milk.
4. Pour the wet ingredients into the dry ingredients and stir just until combined. Be careful not to overmix.
5. Gently fold in the fresh berries.
6. Distribute the batter evenly among the muffin cups.
7. Bake in the preheated oven for 20-25 minutes or until a toothpick inserted into the center of a muffin comes out clean.
8. Allow the muffins to cool in the pan for 5 minutes, then transfer to a wire rack to cool completely.

Nutritional Values (per muffin):
- Calories: 120
- Protein: 4g
- Carbohydrates: 22g
- Dietary Fiber: 4g

Cooking Tip: These muffins freeze well! Store them in an airtight container in the freezer and thaw at room temperature or in the microwave when ready to enjoy.

Recipe 3: Spinach and Mushroom Breakfast Scramble (no oil)

Prep Time: 10 minutes - Cooking Time: 10 minutes - Number of Servings: 4

Ingredients:

- 4 cups fresh spinach, chopped.
- 2 cups mushrooms, sliced (e.g., cremini or white button mushrooms)
- 6 large eggs
- 1/4 cup unsweetened almond milk or any milk of choice
- Salt and pepper to taste.
- 1/2 tsp garlic powder
- 2 green onions, sliced.
- 1/4 cup fresh parsley, chopped.
- Water or vegetable broth (for sautéing)

Instructions:

1. Heat a large non-stick skillet over medium heat. Add a couple of tablespoons of water or vegetable broth.

2. Once heated, add the mushrooms. Sauté until they release their moisture and begin to brown about 4-5 minutes.

3. Add the spinach to the skillet and cook until wilted about 2 minutes.

4. In a bowl, whisk together the eggs, almond milk, garlic powder, salt, and pepper.

5. Pour the egg mixture over the spinach and mushrooms in the skillet. Cook, stirring occasionally, until the eggs are scrambled and fully cooked.

6. Remove from heat and stir in the green onions and fresh parsley.

7. Serve hot with your choice of whole-grain toast or fruit on the side.

Nutritional Values (per serving):
- Calories: 110
- Protein: 9g
- Carbohydrates: 4g
- Dietary Fiber: 1g

Cooking Tip: For added flavor, sprinkle some nutritional yeast on top of the scramble before serving. It gives a cheesy taste without the actual cheese.

Recipe 4: Chilled Melon Soup with Fresh Mint

Prep Time: 15 minutes - Chill Time: 1 hour - Number of Servings: 4

Ingredients:

- 4 cups cantaloupe, cubed (about 1 medium-sized melon)
- 2 cups honeydew melon, cubed.
- Juice of 1 lime
- 1/4 cup fresh mint leaves, plus extra for garnish
- 1 cup unsweetened coconut water
- 1 tbsp honey or maple syrup (optional for added sweetness)
- A pinch of salt

Instructions:

1. In a blender, combine the cantaloupe, honeydew melon, lime juice, fresh mint leaves, coconut water, honey or maple syrup (if using), and salt.

2. Blend until smooth.

3. Taste and adjust sweetness or acidity (with more honey or lime juice) as needed.

4. Pour the soup into a large bowl, cover, and refrigerate for at least 1 hour to chill.

5. Serve cold, garnished with additional fresh mint leaves.

Nutritional Values (per serving):

- Calories: 90

- Protein: 2g

- Carbohydrates: 22g

- Dietary Fiber: 2g

Cooking Tip: For an added touch, serve with a dollop of low-fat Greek yogurt on top or sprinkle with some toasted coconut flakes.

Recipe 5: Whole Grain Toast with Smashed Avocado and Cherry Tomatoes

Prep Time: 10 minutes - Cooking Time: 2-3 minutes (for toasting) - Number of Servings: 4

Ingredients:

- 4 slices of whole-grain bread
- 2 ripe avocados
- 1 cup cherry tomatoes, halved.
- Juice of 1 lemon
- Salt and pepper to taste.
- Red pepper flakes (optional)
- Fresh basil or parsley for garnish (optional)

Instructions:

1. Toast the whole grain bread slices to your desired level of crispiness.

2. While the bread is toasting, cut the avocados in half and remove the pit. Scoop out the flesh into a medium-sized bowl.

3. Add the lemon juice to the avocado and mash using a fork until it's mostly smooth but still has some texture.

4. Season with salt, pepper, and red pepper flakes (if using). Mix well.

5. Once the toast is ready, spread a generous amount of the smashed avocado onto each slice.

6. Top with halved cherry tomatoes.

7. Garnish with fresh basil or parsley if desired.

8. Serve immediately.

Nutritional Values (per serving):

- Calories: 230

- Protein: 7g

- Carbohydrates: 25g

- Dietary Fiber: 9g

Cooking Tip: For a richer flavor, drizzle a tiny bit of extra virgin olive oil on top or sprinkle with some crumbled feta cheese.

Recipe 6: Barley and Vegetable Hash with Fresh Herbs

Prep Time: 10 minutes - Cooking Time: 35-40 minutes - Number of Servings: 4

Ingredients:

- 1 cup pearled barley rinsed and drained.
- 2.5 cups vegetable broth or water
- 1 medium zucchini, diced.
- 1 red bell pepper, diced.
- 1 cup cherry tomatoes, halved.
- 1 small red onion finely chopped.
- 2 garlic cloves, minced.
- 2 tbsp fresh parsley, chopped.
- 1 tbsp fresh basil, chopped.
- Salt and pepper to taste.
- Water or vegetable broth (for sautéing)
- Fresh lemon juice (optional)

Instructions:

1. In a medium-sized pot, combine barley and vegetable broth (or water). Bring to a boil.
2. Reduce heat, cover, and simmer until barley is tender and most of the liquid has been absorbed, about 30 minutes.
3. While the barley is cooking, heat a large skillet over medium heat. Add a splash of water or vegetable broth.
4. Sauté the onion and garlic until translucent, about 3 minutes.
5. Add the zucchini and bell pepper to the skillet. Cook until softened, about 5-7 minutes.
6. Stir in the cherry tomatoes and cook for an additional 2 minutes.
7. Once the barley is done, add it to the skillet with the vegetables. Mix well.
8. Season with salt, pepper, and fresh herbs. Give everything a good stir.
9. Serve hot with a squeeze of fresh lemon juice on top if desired.

Nutritional Values (per serving):

- Calories: 210

- Protein: 6g

- Carbohydrates: 47g

- Dietary Fiber: 10g

Cooking Tip: You can add other veggies of your choice or some canned beans for extra protein. This hash pairs well with a green salad or roasted vegetables.

Recipe 7: Steel-cut oats with Cinnamon, Apple, and Walnuts

Prep Time: 5 minutes - Cooking Time: 25-30 minutes - Number of Servings: 4

Ingredients:

- 1 cup steel-cut oats
- 4 cups water
- 2 medium apples cored and chopped.
- 1 tsp ground cinnamon
- 1/4 cup chopped walnuts.
- 1/4 cup raisins or dried cranberries (optional)
- 12 tbsp maple syrup or honey (optional for added sweetness)
- A pinch of salt

Instructions:

1. In a medium-sized pot, bring water to a boil. Add a pinch of salt.

2. Once boiling, slowly stir in the steel-cut oats.

3. Reduce the heat to a simmer and cook, stirring occasionally, for 20-25 minutes or until the oats have absorbed most of the water and have a creamy consistency.

4. While the oats are cooking, in another skillet over medium heat, add the chopped apples and cook until they begin to soften about 5 minutes.

5. Stir in the cinnamon and continue to cook for another 2 minutes.

6. Once the oats are ready, stir in the apple-cinnamon mixture.

7. Serve the oats in individual bowls. Top with chopped walnuts, raisins, or cranberries if used, and a drizzle of maple syrup or honey if desired.

Nutritional Values (per serving):

- Calories: 235

- Protein: 7g

- Carbohydrates: 39g

- Dietary Fiber: 6g

Cooking Tip: For a creamier texture, you can cook the oats in almond milk or another milk of choice instead of water.

Recipe 8: Broccoli and Red Pepper Egg White Omelette

Prep Time: 10 minutes - Cooking Time: 10 minutes - Number of Servings: 2

Ingredients:

- 1 cup broccoli florets, chopped.
- 1/2 red bell pepper, diced.
- 6 egg whites
- 1/4 cup unsweetened almond milk (or any milk of choice)
- Salt and pepper to taste.
- 1/4 tsp paprika (optional)
- 2 tbsp fresh chives, chopped.
- Water or vegetable broth (for sautéing)

Instructions:

1. Heat a non-stick skillet over medium heat. Add a splash of water or vegetable broth.

2. Sauté the broccoli and red bell pepper until they begin to soften, about 4-5 minutes.

3. In a bowl, whisk together the egg whites, almond milk, salt, pepper, and paprika if using.

4. Pour the egg white mixture over the broccoli and red bell pepper in the skillet. Allow it to set for a couple of minutes.

5. Gently stir the omelet, ensuring it cooks evenly. Once mostly set but still slightly runny on top, flip one side over the other.

6. Cover the skillet and cook for another 2-3 minutes until the omelet is fully set.

7. Serve hot, garnished with fresh chives.

Nutritional Values (per serving):

- Calories: 90

- Protein: 17g

- Carbohydrates: 5g

- Dietary Fiber: 2g

Cooking Tip: For a spicier kick, you can add some diced jalapeño or sprinkle some chili flakes on top. Serve with whole grain toast or a side salad for a complete meal.

Recipe 9: Fresh Fruit Salad with a Splash of Orange Juice

Prep Time: 15 minutes - Cooking Time: None - Number of Servings: 4

Ingredients:

- 1 cup strawberries hulled and halved.
- 1 cup blueberries
- 1 cup pineapple chunks
- 1 cup kiwi peeled and sliced.
- 1 cup mango peeled and diced.
- Juice of 2 oranges

Instructions:

1. In a large bowl, combine strawberries, blueberries, pineapple, kiwi, and mango.

2. Squeeze the juice from the two oranges, ensuring there are no seeds, and pour over the fruit.

3. Gently toss the fruit to mix well and ensure it's coated with the orange juice.

4. Chill in the refrigerator for about 10 minutes before serving to allow the flavors to meld.

5. Serve in individual bowls with a spoonful of orange juice from the bottom of the bowl drizzled on top.

Nutritional Values (per serving):

- Calories: 110

- Protein: 2g

- Carbohydrates: 28g

- Dietary Fiber: 4g

Cooking Tip: You can add a sprinkle of chia seeds or flax seeds on top for added texture and nutrition. Also, feel free to mix and match fruits based on seasonality and personal preferences.

Recipe 10: Rye Pancakes Topped with Stewed Berries (no added sugars)

Prep Time: 15 minutes - Cooking Time: 20 minutes - Number of Servings: 4 (about 8-10 pancakes)

Ingredients:
- 1 cup rye flour
- 1 tsp baking powder
- 1/2 tsp baking soda
- 1/4 tsp salt
- 1 cup buttermilk (or almond milk with a tsp of lemon juice)
- 1 large egg
- 1 tsp pure vanilla extract
- 2 cups mixed berries (such as blueberries, raspberries, blackberries)
- 1/2 cup water
- 1 tbsp lemon zest

Instructions:
1. Start by preparing the stewed berries. In a saucepan, combine mixed berries, water, and lemon zest. Bring to a simmer over medium heat and allow to cook until berries break down and form a sauce, about 10-12 minutes. Set it aside and keep warm.
2. In a mixing bowl, whisk together rye flour, baking powder, baking soda, and salt.
3. In a separate bowl, combine buttermilk, egg, and vanilla extract.
4. Pour the wet ingredients into the dry ingredients and mix until just combined.
5. Preheat a non-stick skillet or griddle over medium heat.
6. Ladle about 1/4 cup of batter for each pancake onto the skillet. Cook until bubbles form on the surface, then flip and cook for another 1-2 minutes on the other side.
7. Repeat with the remaining batter.
8. Serve pancakes warm, topped with stewed berries.

Nutritional Values (per serving):
- Calories: 210
- Protein: 7g
- Carbohydrates: 40g
- Dietary Fiber: 7g

Cooking Tip: If you desire a sweeter taste, you can add a drizzle of pure maple syrup or a dollop of low-fat Greek yogurt on top of the pancakes.

Recipe 11: Zucchini and Corn Breakfast Burritos (whole grain tortillas)

Prep Time: 15 minutes - Cooking Time: 20 minutes - Number of Servings: 4

Ingredients:
- 4 whole grain tortillas
- 2 zucchinis, diced.
- 1 cup corn kernels (fresh or frozen)
- 1 red bell pepper, diced.
- 1/2 red onion finely chopped.
- 4 large eggs, whisked.
- 1/4 cup fresh cilantro, chopped.
- Salt and pepper to taste.
- 1 avocado, sliced.
- Water or vegetable broth (for sautéing)
- Salsa or hot sauce (optional)

Instructions:
1. In a large skillet, heat a splash of water or vegetable broth over medium heat.
2. Add red onion, zucchini, and bell pepper. Sauté until they begin to soften, about 4-5 minutes.
3. Add corn kernels and continue to cook for another 3 minutes.
4. Push the vegetables to one side of the skillet, and on the other side, pour in the whisked eggs. Cook, stirring frequently, until the eggs are scrambled and cooked through.
5. Combine the vegetables and scrambled eggs, mixing well. Season with salt and pepper.
6. Warm the whole grain tortillas in a dry skillet or microwave for about 10-15 seconds.
7. Lay out a tortilla and place a quarter of the zucchini-corn-egg mixture in the center. Top with avocado slices and fresh cilantro.
8. Roll up the tortilla, tucking in the ends as you go.
9. Serve immediately with salsa or hot sauce if desired.

Nutritional Values (per serving):

- Calories: 290

- Protein: 11g

- Carbohydrates: 37g

- Dietary Fiber: 8g

Cooking Tip: For added protein, sprinkle some black beans or cheese into the burrito before rolling.

Recipe 12: Banana and Blueberry Smoothie with Chia Seeds (no added sugars)

Prep Time: 10 minutes - Cooking Time: None - Number of Servings: 2

Ingredients:

1. 2 ripe bananas
2. 1 cup blueberries (fresh or frozen)
3. 2 tbsp chia seeds
4. 1 1/2 cups unsweetened almond milk (or any milk of choice)
5. 1/2 tsp vanilla extract
6. A pinch of ground cinnamon (optional)
7. Ice cubes (optional)

Instructions:

1. In a blender, combine bananas, blueberries, chia seeds, almond milk, vanilla extract, and ground cinnamon if using.

2. If you prefer a colder smoothie, you can also add a few ice cubes.

3. Blend on high until smooth and creamy.

4. Pour into glasses and serve immediately.

Nutritional Values (per serving):

- Calories: 190

- Protein: 5g

- Carbohydrates: 37g

- Dietary Fiber: 9g

Cooking Tip: For added nutrition, consider blending in a handful of spinach or kale. It won't significantly change the taste but will boost the smoothie's nutritional content.

Recipe 13: Lentil and Kale Morning Stew

Prep Time: 10 minutes - Cooking Time: 35-40 minutes - Number of Servings: 4

Ingredients:

- 1 cup dried green lentils rinsed and drained.
- 4 cups vegetable broth or water
- 2 cups kale chopped and stems removed.
- 1 medium onion finely chopped.
- 2 garlic cloves, minced.
- 1 carrot, diced.
- 1 celery stalk, diced.
- 1 tsp ground turmeric
- 1/2 tsp ground cumin
- Salt and pepper to taste.
- Juice of half a lemon
- 2 tbsp fresh parsley, chopped.
- Water or vegetable broth (for sautéing)

Instructions:

1. In a large pot, sauté the onion, carrot, and celery with a splash of water or vegetable broth over medium heat until softened, about 5 minutes.
2. Add the garlic and continue to sauté for another 2 minutes.
3. Stir in the lentils, turmeric, cumin, and vegetable broth or water. Bring to a boil.
4. Reduce the heat, cover, and let simmer for about 25 minutes or until lentils are tender.
5. Stir in the chopped kale and continue to cook until wilted about 5 minutes.
6. Season with salt, pepper, and lemon juice. Mix well.
7. Serve hot, garnished with fresh parsley.

Nutritional Values (per serving):

- Calories: 210

- Protein: 13g

- Carbohydrates: 37g

- Dietary Fiber: 16g

Cooking Tip: For a richer flavor, consider adding a bay leaf or some smoked paprika to the stew while it's simmering.

Recipe 14: Pineapple and Mango Overnight Oats with Almond Slivers

Prep Time: 15 minutes - Chill Time: 8 hours (overnight) - Number of Servings: 4

Ingredients:

- 1 cup rolled oats.
- 2 cups unsweetened almond milk (or any milk of choice)
- 1 cup pineapple chunks
- 1 cup mango chunks
- 2 tbsp chia seeds
- 1 tsp pure vanilla extract
- 1/4 cup almond slivers
- 2 tbsp shredded unsweetened coconut (optional)
- A pinch of salt

Instructions:

1. In a large mixing bowl, combine the rolled oats, chia seeds, vanilla extract, and salt.

2. Add the almond milk and stir until everything is well combined.

3. Fold in the pineapple and mango chunks.

4. Divide the mixture among 4 mason jars or airtight containers.

5. Seal the jars or containers and place them in the refrigerator overnight.

6. The next morning, give the oats a good stir. If they're too thick, you can add a splash of almond milk to achieve your desired consistency.

7. Top with almond slivers and shredded coconut if using.

8. Enjoy cold directly from the jar or container.

Nutritional Values (per serving):

- Calories: 230

- Protein: 6g

- Carbohydrates: 37g

- Dietary Fiber: 8g

Cooking Tip: Feel free to add a drizzle of honey or maple syrup if you prefer your overnight oats to be a bit sweeter. You can also experiment with other fruits or nuts to vary the flavors.

Chapter 7: Lunch Recipes

Welcome to Chapter 7 of *"The Pritikin Diet for Seniors: The Complete Guide to Weight Loss and Improved Health for Seniors."* When it comes to lunchtime, it's an opportunity to refuel and recharge, ensuring that you stay on track with your weight management goals and overall well-being. In this chapter, we have carefully selected a variety of nutritious lunch recipes specifically tailored for seniors.

Our lunch recipes are meticulously crafted to provide the energy you need to power through the day while keeping an eye on calorie counts. We understand the importance of satisfaction during lunchtime. These recipes excel in both taste and nutrition.

You will find an array of options that incorporate proteins, whole grains, and a colorful abundance of vegetables. These choices are designed to support weight management. Whether you prefer salads bursting with flavors, hearty soups, or creative sandwich ideas, this chapter offers something for every palate and dietary preference.

While exploring these lunch recipes, you will discover that maintaining a body weight can be more enjoyable than a chore. These recipes showcase the idea that nutritious eating can contribute significantly to your longevity while being delightful at the time.

So, let us embark on this adventure together and make lunchtime a delicious and healthy part of your routine.

In this section, you'll discover some recipes that not only provide nourishment to your body but also help you maintain a healthy weight. The best part is they taste delicious!

Chapter 7: Pritikin Lunch Delights

15. Mixed Bean Salad with Fresh Cilantro and Lime Dressing

16. Grilled Veggie Wraps in Whole Wheat Tortillas with Hummus Spread

17. Lentil Soup with Spinach and Diced Tomatoes

18. Quinoa Tabouli with Fresh Parsley and Lemon Zest

19. Grilled Portobello Mushrooms Stuffed with Spinach and Roasted Peppers

20. Spicy Chickpea and Kale Stew

21. Cold Cucumber and Dill Soup with a Touch of Garlic

22. Whole Grain Pasta Salad with Mixed Vegetables and Lemon Vinaigrette

23. Roasted Beet and Orange Salad on a Bed of Arugula

24. Zucchini Noodles Tossed in Fresh Tomato and Basil Sauce

25. Eggplant Roll-Ups with a Spinach and Ricotta (low-fat) Filling

26. Stuffed Bell Peppers with Brown Rice and Black Beans

27. Tofu and Broccoli Stir-Fry over Brown Rice (minimal oil)

28. Fresh Spring Rolls with Vegetables and a Tangy Tamarind Dipping Sauce

Recipe 15: Mixed Bean Salad with Fresh Cilantro and Lime Dressing

Prep Time: 15 minutes - Chill Time: 1 hour - Number of Servings: 4

Ingredients:

- 1 cup cooked black beans (rinsed and drained if using canned)
- 1 cup cooked kidney beans (rinsed and drained if using canned)
- 1 cup cooked chickpeas (rinsed and drained if using released)
- 1 red bell pepper, diced.
- 1/2 red onion finely chopped.
- 1/4 cup fresh cilantro, chopped.
- Zest and juice of 1 lime
- 2 tbsp extra virgin olive oil or avocado oil
- 1 garlic clove, minced.
- Salt and pepper to taste.

Instructions:

1. In a large mixing bowl, combine the black beans, kidney beans, chickpeas, red bell pepper, and red onion.

2. In a separate small bowl, whisk together the lime zest, lime juice, olive oil, minced garlic, salt, and pepper to create the dressing.

3. Pour the dressing over the bean mixture and toss to coat evenly.

4. Fold in the fresh cilantro.

5. Cover the salad and refrigerate for at least 1 hour to let the flavors meld.

6. Toss again before serving and adjust seasonings if needed.

Nutritional Values (per serving):

- Calories: 260

- Protein: 12g

- Carbohydrates: 39g

- Dietary Fiber: 12g

Cooking Tip: This salad can be served on its own or over a bed of fresh greens. You can also add diced avocado for creaminess and additional healthy fats.

Recipe 16: Grilled Veggie Wraps in Whole Wheat Tortillas with Hummus Spread

Prep Time: 20 minutes - Cooking Time: 10 minutes - Number of Servings: 4

Ingredients:
- 4 whole wheat tortillas
- 1 cup hummus (storebought or homemade)
- 1 zucchini, sliced lengthwise into thin strips.
- 1 red bell pepper, sliced into strips.
- 1 yellow bell pepper, sliced into strips.
- 1 red onion, sliced into rings.
- 1 cup baby spinach leaves
- Water or vegetable broth (for grilling)
- Salt and pepper to taste.

Instructions:
1. Preheat a grill or grill pan over medium-high heat.
2. Lightly brush the zucchini slices, bell pepper strips, and red onion rings with water or vegetable broth. Season with salt and pepper.
3. Grill the vegetables for about 3-4 minutes on each side or until they have nice grill marks and are slightly tender.
4. Remove the vegetables from the grill and set aside.
5. Lay out a whole wheat tortilla and spread a generous amount of hummus over the surface.
6. Place a handful of baby spinach leaves in the center of the tortilla.
7. Add a portion of the grilled vegetables on top of the spinach.
8. Roll up the tortilla, folding in the sides as you go, to create a wrap.
9. Repeat with the remaining tortillas and ingredients.
10. Slice each wrap in half diagonally and serve.

Nutritional Values (per serving):

- Calories: 280

- Protein: 9g

- Carbohydrates: 44g

- Dietary Fiber: 7g

Cooking Tip: For added flavor, sprinkle some feta cheese or drizzle a bit of balsamic reduction inside the wrap before rolling.

Recipe 17: Lentil Soup with Spinach and Diced Tomatoes

Prep Time: 15 minutes - Cooking Time: 40 minutes - Number of Servings: 4-6

Ingredients:

- 1 cup dried green lentils rinsed and drained.
- 6 cups low-sodium vegetable broth
- 1 can (14.5 oz) diced tomatoes, undrained.
- 2 cups fresh spinach, chopped.
- 1 medium onion, diced.
- 2 garlic cloves, minced.
- 2 carrots, diced.
- 2 celery stalks, diced.
- 1 tsp ground cumin
- 1/2 tsp ground turmeric
- Salt and pepper to taste.
- Juice of 1 lemon
- 2 tbsp fresh parsley, chopped (for garnish)
- Water or vegetable broth (for sautéing)

Instructions:

1. In a large pot, sauté the onion, carrots, and celery with a splash of water or vegetable broth over medium heat until softened, about 5 minutes.
2. Add the minced garlic and sauté for an additional 2 minutes.
3. Stir in the lentils, cumin, turmeric, and vegetable broth. Increase the heat and bring the mixture to a boil.
4. Once boiling, reduce the heat, cover, and simmer for about 30 minutes or until the lentils are tender.
5. Add the diced tomatoes (with their juices) and fresh spinach. Stir well and continue to simmer for an additional 5-7 minutes.
6. Season the soup with salt, pepper, and lemon juice. Adjust the seasonings to your liking.
7. Serve hot, garnished with fresh parsley.

Nutritional Values (per serving):

- Calories: 190

- Protein: 11g

- Carbohydrates: 32g

- Dietary Fiber: 14g

Cooking Tip: For added richness, you can swirl in a spoonful of low-fat Greek yogurt or a drizzle of extra virgin olive oil before serving.

Recipe 18: Quinoa Tabouli with Fresh Parsley and Lemon Zest

Prep Time: 20 minutes - Cooking Time: 15 minutes - Chill Time: 1 hour - Number of Servings: 4-6

Ingredients:

- 1 cup quinoa rinsed and drained.
- 2 cups water
- 2 cups fresh parsley finely chopped.
- 1 cup cherry tomatoes, halved.
- 1/2 cucumber, diced.
- 4 green onions, sliced.
- Zest and juice of 2 lemons
- 2 tbsp extra virgin olive oil
- Salt and pepper to taste.

Instructions:

1. In a medium pot, bring the water to a boil. Add a pinch of salt and the rinsed quinoa.

2. Reduce the heat to low, cover, and simmer for about 12-15 minutes, or until quinoa is tender and the water is absorbed. Remove from heat and fluff with a fork.

3. Transfer the cooked quinoa to a large mixing bowl and let it cool to room temperature.

4. Once cooled, add the parsley, cherry tomatoes, cucumber, and green onions to the bowl.

5. In a separate small bowl, whisk together the lemon zest, lemon juice, olive oil, salt, and pepper to create the dressing.

6. Pour the dressing over the quinoa mixture and toss to combine everything thoroughly.

7. Cover the tabouli and refrigerate for at least 1 hour to let the flavors meld.

8. Serve chilled, adjusting seasonings if necessary.

Nutritional Values (per serving):

- Calories: 180

- Protein: 5g

- Carbohydrates: 27g

- Dietary Fiber: 4g

Cooking Tip: Traditional tabouli uses bulgur wheat, but quinoa is a protein-rich and gluten-free alternative. If you prefer a bit more zest, you can add a finely diced jalapeño pepper.

Recipe 19: Grilled Portobello Mushrooms Stuffed with Spinach and Roasted Peppers

Prep Time: 20 minutes - Cooking Time: 15 minutes - Number of Servings: 4

Ingredients:

- 4 large portobello mushrooms, stems removed and cleaned.
- 2 cups fresh spinach, chopped.
- 1 cup roasted red bell peppers, chopped.
- 2 garlic cloves, minced.
- 1/4 cup low-fat ricotta cheese or dairy-free alternative
- Salt and pepper to taste.
- 1 tbsp fresh basil, chopped (for garnish)
- Water or vegetable broth (for sautéing)

Instructions:

1. Preheat your grill or grill pan to medium heat.

2. In a large skillet over medium heat, sauté garlic in a splash of water or vegetable broth until fragrant, about 1-2 minutes.

3. Add the chopped spinach and cook until wilted, about 3-4 minutes.

4. Stir in the roasted red bell peppers and cook for another 2 minutes.

5. Remove from heat and mix in the ricotta cheese until well combined. Season with salt and pepper.

6. Stuff each portobello mushroom cap with an equal portion of the spinach and roasted pepper mixture.

7. Place the stuffed mushrooms on the grill and cook for about 7 minutes on each side or until the mushrooms are tender and slightly charred.

8. Serve hot, garnished with fresh basil.

Nutritional Values (per serving):

- Calories: 110

- Protein: 6g

- Carbohydrates: 14g

- Dietary Fiber: 3g

Cooking Tip: These grilled portobello mushrooms can be served with a side of quinoa salad or grilled vegetables for a complete meal. If desired, you can sprinkle some crumbled feta cheese on top before grilling.

Recipe 20: Spicy Chickpea and Kale Stew

Prep Time: 15 minutes - Cooking Time: 30 minutes - Number of Servings: 4

Ingredients:

- 2 cups chickpeas (cooked or rinsed and drained if using canned)
- 4 cups chopped kale; stems removed.
- 1 medium onion, diced.
- 2 garlic cloves, minced.
- 1 can (14.5 oz) diced tomatoes, undrained.
- 4 cups vegetable broth or water
- 1 tsp ground cumin
- 1/2 tsp ground coriander
- 1/4 tsp chili flakes (adjust to your heat preference)
- 1 tbsp extra-virgin olive oil or avocado oil
- Salt and pepper to taste
- Juice of 1 lemon
- Fresh cilantro or parsley for garnish

Instructions:

1. In a large pot, heat the olive oil over medium heat. Add the diced onion and sauté until translucent, about 4 minutes.
2. Add the minced garlic, ground cumin, ground coriander, and chili flakes. Continue to sauté for another 2 minutes until fragrant.
3. Stir in the diced tomatoes (with their juices) and the chickpeas. Mix well.
4. Add the vegetable broth or water and bring the mixture to a boil.
5. Once boiling, reduce the heat to low, cover, and let simmer for about 20 minutes.
6. Add the chopped kale and continue to cook until wilted, about 5 minutes.
7. Season the stew with salt, pepper, and lemon juice. Adjust the seasonings to taste.
8. Serve hot, garnished with fresh cilantro or parsley.

Nutritional Values (per serving):

- Calories: 240

- Protein: 11g

- Carbohydrates: 38g

- Dietary Fiber: 9g

Cooking Tip: For a heartier meal, you can add diced potatoes or sweet potatoes at the same time as the tomatoes and chickpeas. This stew pairs wonderfully with a slice of whole-grain bread or a side salad.

Recipe 21: Cold Cucumber and Dill Soup with a Touch of Garlic

Prep Time: 15 minutes - Chill Time: 2 hours - Number of Servings: 4

Ingredients:

- 2 large cucumbers, peeled, seeded, and roughly chopped.
- 2 cups low-fat plain yogurt or dairy-free yogurt alternative
- 2 garlic cloves, minced.
- 3 tbsp fresh dill, chopped.
- 1 tbsp lemon juice
- Salt and pepper to taste.
- 1 tbsp olive oil (optional for drizzling)
- Fresh dill sprigs for garnish

Instructions:

1. In a blender or food processor, combine the chopped cucumbers, yogurt, minced garlic, chopped dill, and lemon juice. Blend until smooth.

2. Season the soup with salt and pepper to taste. Adjust the seasonings according to your preference.

3. Transfer the soup to a bowl, cover it, and chill in the refrigerator for at least 2 hours.

4. Before serving, give the soup a good stir and adjust the consistency with a bit of cold water or additional yogurt if it's too thick.

5. Ladle the soup into individual bowls. Drizzle with a touch of olive oil if desired, and garnish with fresh dill sprigs.

6. Serve cold.

Nutritional Values (per serving):

- Calories: 90 (without olive oil)

- Protein: 5g

- Carbohydrates: 12g

- Dietary Fiber: 1g

Cooking Tip: This refreshing soup is perfect for hot summer days. For a more pronounced garlic flavor, you can add an extra clove. You can also garnish with finely diced cucumbers for added texture.

Recipe 22: Whole Grain Pasta Salad with Mixed Vegetables and Lemon Vinaigrette

Prep Time: 20 minutes - Cooking Time: 10 minutes - Chill Time: 1 hour - Number of Servings: 4-6

Ingredients:

- 2 cups whole grain pasta (penne, fusilli, or any shape you prefer)
- 1 cup cherry tomatoes, halved.
- 1 bell pepper (any color), diced.
- 1/2 cucumber, diced.
- 1/4 red onion finely sliced.
- 1/4 cup fresh basil, chopped.
- 1/4 cup fresh parsley, chopped.

Lemon Vinaigrette:

Zest and juice of 1 lemon
2 tbsp extra-virgin olive oil or avocado oil
1 garlic clove, minced.
Salt and pepper to taste.

Instructions:

1. Cook the whole grain pasta according to the package instructions until al dente. Drain and rinse under cold water to cool and stop the cooking process.
2. In a large mixing bowl, combine the cooked pasta, cherry tomatoes, bell pepper, cucumber, red onion, basil, and parsley.
3. For the vinaigrette: In a small bowl, whisk together the lemon zest, lemon juice, olive oil, minced garlic, salt, and pepper.
4. Pour the vinaigrette over the pasta salad and toss to coat all the ingredients evenly.
5. Cover the salad and refrigerate for at least 1 hour to let the flavors meld.
6. Before serving, give the salad a good toss and adjust seasonings if needed.

Nutritional Values (per serving):

- Calories: 220

- Protein: 7g

- Carbohydrates: 38g

- Dietary Fiber: 6g

Cooking Tip: This versatile pasta salad is perfect for picnics and gatherings. You can add other ingredients like olives, feta cheese, or grilled chicken for added flavor and variety.

Recipe 23: Roasted Beet and Orange Salad on a Bed of Arugula

Prep Time: 20 minutes - Cooking Time: 45 minutes (for roasting beets) - Number of Servings: 4

Ingredients:

- 3 medium beets scrubbed clean.
- 2 large oranges peeled and segmented.
- 4 cups arugula
- 1/4 cup red onion thinly sliced.
- 1/4 cup crumbled feta cheese (optional)
- 2 tbsp fresh mint, chopped.
- 2 tbsp extra-virgin olive oil
- 1 tbsp balsamic vinegar
- Salt and pepper to taste.

Instructions:

1. Preheat your oven to 400°F (200°C).

2. Wrap each beet individually in aluminum foil and place them on a baking sheet.

3. Roast in the preheated oven for about 45 minutes or until the beets are tender when pierced with a fork.

4. Once done, remove them from the oven and let them cool. Once cooled, peel and slice the beets.

5. In a large salad bowl, combine the arugula, sliced beets, orange segments, and red onion.

6. In a small bowl, whisk together the olive oil, balsamic vinegar, salt, and pepper to make the dressing.

7. Pour the dressing over the salad and toss gently to combine.

8. Garnish the salad with crumbled feta cheese (if using) and fresh mint.

9. Serve immediately.

Nutritional Values (per serving):

- Calories: 180 (without feta)

- Protein: 3g

- Carbohydrates: 25g

- Dietary Fiber: 5g

Cooking Tip: The natural sweetness of roasted beets pairs wonderfully with the citrusy flavor of oranges. If you're short on time, you can use pre-cooked beets available at many grocery stores.

Recipe 24: Zucchini Noodles Tossed in Fresh Tomato and Basil Sauce

Prep Time: 15 minutes - Cooking Time: 10 minutes - Number of Servings: 4

Ingredients:

- 4 medium zucchinis, spiralized into noodles
- 2 cups cherry tomatoes, halved.
- 3 garlic cloves, minced.
- 1/4 cup fresh basil leaves, chopped.
- 1/4 cup grated Parmesan cheese or nutritional yeast (for a dairy-free alternative)
- 2 tbsp extra virgin olive oil or avocado oil
- Salt and pepper to taste.
- Red pepper flakes (optional for added heat)
- Water or vegetable broth (for sautéing)

Instructions:

1. In a large skillet, heat a splash of water or vegetable broth over medium heat. Add the minced garlic and sauté until fragrant, about 1-2 minutes.
2. Add the halved cherry tomatoes to the skillet. Cook for about 5 minutes or until the tomatoes start to break down and release their juices.
3. Add the zucchini noodles to the skillet, tossing to combine with the tomatoes and garlic. Cook for another 3-4 minutes, just until the noodles are heated through but still retain some crunch.
4. Remove from heat and stir in the fresh basil, olive oil, and Parmesan cheese or nutritional yeast. Season with salt, pepper, and red pepper flakes if used.
5. Toss everything together until well combined and the noodles are coated with the sauce.
6. Serve immediately, garnishing with additional cheese or basil if desired.

Nutritional Values (per serving):

- Calories: 150 (with Parmesan cheese)

- Protein: 6g

- Carbohydrates: 12g

- Dietary Fiber: 4g

Cooking Tip: Zucchini noodles (often called "zoodles") are a great low-carb alternative to traditional pasta. To prevent them from getting too watery, it's important not to overcook them.

Recipe 25: Eggplant Roll-Ups with Spinach and Ricotta (low-fat) Filling

Prep Time: 20 minutes - Cooking Time: 40 minutes - Number of Servings: 4

Ingredients:
- 2 medium eggplants, sliced lengthwise into 1/4-inch-thick strips.
- 1 cup low-fat ricotta cheese
- 2 cups fresh spinach, chopped.
- 2 garlic cloves, minced.
- 1/4 cup grated Parmesan cheese
- 1 egg (lightly beaten)
- 1 cup marinara sauce (no sugar added)
- Salt and pepper to taste.
- Olive oil or avocado oil spray
- Fresh basil leaves (for garnish)

Instructions:
1. Preheat your oven to 375°F (190°C).
2. Lightly spray a baking sheet with olive oil or avocado oil. Lay the eggplant slices on the sheet in a single layer and lightly spray the tops. Season with salt and pepper.
3. Bake the eggplant slices in the preheated oven for about 15 minutes or until they are soft and pliable. Please remove it from the oven and let it cool.
4. While the eggplant is baking, heat a skillet over medium heat. Add the chopped spinach and minced garlic, sautéing until the spinach is wilted. Remove from heat and let cool.
5. In a mixing bowl, combine the ricotta cheese, spinach mixture, grated Parmesan cheese, and beaten egg. Mix until well combined and season with salt and pepper.
6. Spread a thin layer of marinara sauce on the bottom of a baking dish.
7. Place a spoonful of the ricotta-spinach mixture on one end of each eggplant slice. Roll up the slice and place it seam-side down in the baking dish. Repeat with the remaining pieces.
8. Pour the remaining marinara sauce over the eggplant roll-ups.
9. Bake in the oven for 20-25 minutes or until the sauce is bubbly and the roll-ups are heated through.
10. Garnish with fresh basil leaves before serving.

Nutritional Values (per serving):
- Calories: 180
- Protein: 11g
- Carbohydrates: 20g
- Dietary Fiber: 8g

Cooking Tip: For added flavor, sprinkle some mozzarella cheese on top of the roll-ups before baking. This will create a deliciously melty and golden top layer.

Recipe 26: Stuffed Bell Peppers with Brown Rice and Black Beans

Prep Time: 25 minutes - Cooking Time: 40 minutes - Number of Servings: 4

Ingredients:

- 4 large bell peppers (any color), tops removed, and seeds discarded.
- 1 cup cooked brown rice.
- 1 cup cooked black beans (rinsed and drained if using canned)
- 1 cup corn kernels (fresh, frozen, or canned)
- 1 medium onion finely diced.
- 2 garlic cloves, minced.
- 1 tsp ground cumin
- 1 tsp smoked paprika.
- Salt and pepper to taste.
- 1 1/2 cups tomato sauce (no sugar added)
- 1 tbsp extra virgin olive oil or avocado oil
- Fresh cilantro or parsley for garnish

Instructions:

1. Preheat your oven to 375°F (190°C).
2. In a large skillet, heat the olive oil over medium heat. Add the diced onion and sauté until translucent, about 4 minutes.
3. Add the minced garlic, cumin, and smoked paprika. Continue to sauté for another 2 minutes.
4. Stir in the black beans, corn, and brown rice. Mix until all ingredients are well combined. Season with salt and pepper.
5. Pour half of the tomato sauce into the bottom of a baking dish.
6. Stuff each bell pepper with the rice and bean mixture, pressing down gently to pack the filling.
7. Place the stuffed bell peppers in the baking dish. Pour the remaining tomato sauce over the top.
8. Cover the baking dish with aluminum foil and bake in the preheated oven for 35-40 minutes or until the peppers are tender.
9. Garnish with fresh cilantro or parsley before serving.

Nutritional Values (per serving):

- Calories: 260

- Protein: 8g

- Carbohydrates: 49g

- Dietary Fiber: 9g

Cooking Tip: For a cheesy variation, sprinkle some shredded cheese on top of the stuffed peppers during the last 10 minutes of baking.

Recipe 27: Tofu and Broccoli Stir-Fry over Brown Rice (minimal oil)

Prep Time: 20 minutes - Cooking Time: 20 minutes - Number of Servings: 4

Ingredients:
- 1 block (14 oz) firm tofu, drained, pressed, and cut into cubes.
- 4 cups broccoli florets
- 2 bell peppers (any color), sliced into strips.
- 1 carrot, julienned
- 3 garlic cloves, minced.
- 2 tbsp low sodium soy sauce or tamari
- 1 tbsp rice vinegar
- 1 tsp sesame oil
- 1 tsp chili flakes (optional, for added heat)
- 2 tsp cornstarch mixed with 2 tbsp water.
- 1 cup brown rice, cooked according to package instructions.
- Green onions, sliced (for garnish)
- Water or vegetable broth (for sautéing)

Instructions:
1. In a large wok or non-stick skillet, heat a splash of water or vegetable broth over medium-high heat. Add the tofu cubes and stir-fry until lightly golden, about 4-5 minutes. Remove tofu from the skillet and set aside.

2. In the same skillet, add more water or broth as needed, then stir-fry the broccoli, bell peppers, and carrot until they begin to soften, about 5 minutes.
3. Add the minced garlic to the skillet and stir-fry for an additional minute.
4. Return the tofu to the skillet. In a small bowl, combine the soy sauce, rice vinegar, sesame oil, and chili flakes if using. Pour this mixture over the tofu and vegetables.
5. Stir the cornstarch and water mixture once more and add it to the skillet. Stir everything well, ensuring the tofu and vegetables are coated with the sauce. Continue to cook for another 2-3 minutes or until the sauce has thickened.
6. Serve the tofu and broccoli stir-fry over cooked brown rice and garnish with sliced green onions.

Nutritional Values (per serving):
- Calories: 300
- Protein: 18g
- Carbohydrates: 44g
- Dietary Fiber: 7g

Cooking Tip: For extra flavor and a touch of sweetness, you can add a tablespoon of hoisin sauce or maple syrup to the soy sauce mixture.

Recipe 28: Fresh Spring Rolls with Vegetables and a Tangy Tamarind Dipping Sauce

Prep Time: 30 minutes - Number of Servings: 4 (2 rolls per serving)

Ingredients:

- 8 rice paper wrappers
- 2 cups lettuce, shredded.
- 1 cucumber, julienned
- 1 carrot, julienned
- 1 red bell pepper thinly sliced.
- 1 cup fresh cilantro leaves
- 1 cup fresh mint leaves

Tangy Tamarind Dipping Sauce:

- 2 tbsp tamarind paste
- 2 tbsp low-sodium soy sauce or tamari
- 1 tbsp rice vinegar
- 1 tbsp maple syrup or agave nectar
- 1 garlic clove, minced.
- 1 tsp ginger, grated.
- 1 tsp sesame oil
- Chili flakes (optional, to taste)

Instructions:

1. For the Dipping Sauce: In a small bowl, combine all the ingredients for the dipping sauce and whisk well until blended. Adjust the seasonings according to your preference and set aside.

2. Prepare a large bowl of warm water. Dip a rice paper wrapper into the water for about 10-15 seconds until it softens slightly. Lay the wrapper flat on a clean surface.

3. Place a bit of the shredded lettuce on the bottom third of the rice paper wrapper. Top with some of the julienned cucumber, carrot, bell pepper slices, cilantro, and mint.

4. Fold the sides of the rice paper wrapper inwards, then roll the wrapper up tightly from the bottom, enclosing the filling. Place the finished roll on a plate and cover it with a damp cloth to keep it moist. Repeat with the remaining ingredients.

5. Serve the fresh spring rolls with the tangy tamarind dipping sauce.

Nutritional Values (per serving):

- Calories: 110
- Protein: 3g
- Carbohydrates: 25g
- Dietary Fiber: 3g

Cooking Tip: These fresh spring rolls are versatile. Feel free to add cooked shrimp, grilled chicken, or tofu strips for added protein. You can also play around with different herbs and vegetables according to your preference.

Chapter 8: Main Course Recipes

Welcome to Chapter 8 of "***The Pritikin Diet for Seniors: The Complete Guide to Weight Loss and Improved Health for Seniors***." In this chapter, we have a collection of recipes that will elevate your dining experience. These recipes go beyond satisfying your taste buds: they also focus on nourishing your body and helping you achieve your weight management goals.

We understand that dinner holds a place in your day, and these recipes have been carefully created to strike a balance between flavor and nutrition. Each dish is designed to provide you with the nutrients you need for well-being while keeping calorie intake in check.

From mouthwatering protein options to delicious choices, we offer a wide range of dishes to cater to different dietary preferences. Whether you enjoy comfort foods, crave flavors, or prefer inventive and health-conscious creations, this chapter has something for everyone.

With the Pritikin approach, we emphasize using ingredients, lean proteins, and an abundance of vegetables in every meal. Our goal is to ensure that each dish not only pleases your taste buds but also contributes positively to your long-term health and well-being.

Come along with us on this journey as we delve into main course recipes that will make healthy eating a delightful and long-lasting part of your lifestyle. These delectable dishes will show you that attaining and sustaining a weight can be an enjoyable and fulfilling experience.

Chapter 8: Pritikin Main Course Delights

29. Grilled Lemon-Herb Tilapia with Asparagus Spears

30. Stuffed Acorn Squash with Quinoa, Cranberries, and Spinach

31. Chickpea and Vegetable Curry over Brown Rice

32. Spaghetti Squash Primavera with Fresh Vegetable Medley

33. Grilled Eggplant and Tomato Stacks with Basil Drizzle

34. Lentil and Vegetable Shepherd's Pie Topped with Cauliflower Mash

35. Barley Risotto with Mushrooms and Green Peas

36. Black Bean and Corn Stuffed Poblano Peppers

37. Steamed Cod with Ginger and Scallion Sauce

38. Turmeric and Vegetable Couscous with Roasted Chickpeas

39. Seared Tofu Steaks with Broccoli and Peanut Sauce (low-fat version)

40. Vegetable Paella with Saffron and Artichokes

41. Lemon-Pepper Roasted Brussels Sprouts and Tempeh Bowl

42. Moroccan Vegetable and Chickpea Tagine

These main course recipes align with the principles of the Pritikin Diet, combining wholesome ingredients with flavorful herbs and spices for a heart-healthy and delicious dining experience.

Recipe 29: Grilled Lemon-Herb Tilapia with Asparagus Spears

Prep Time: 15 minutes - Cooking Time: 10 minutes - Number of Servings: 4

Ingredients:

- 4 tilapia fillets (about 56 oz each)
- 1 bunch asparagus spears, trimmed.
- Zest and juice of 2 lemons
- 2 garlic cloves, minced.
- 2 tbsp fresh dill, chopped.
- 2 tbsp fresh parsley, chopped.
- Salt and pepper to taste.
- Olive oil or avocado oil spray

Instructions:

1. Preheat your grill or grill pan to medium-high heat.

2. In a small bowl, mix together lemon zest, lemon juice, minced garlic, dill, and parsley. Season with a pinch of salt and pepper.

3. Lightly spray the tilapia fillets and asparagus spears with olive or avocado oil.

4. Place the tilapia fillets and asparagus spears on the grill. Cook the asparagus for about 4-5 minutes, turning occasionally, until they are slightly charred and tender. Cook the tilapia for about 3-4 minutes per side or until it easily flakes with a fork.

5. During the last minute of grilling, brush the tilapia fillets with the lemon-herb mixture.

6. Once cooked, remove the tilapia and asparagus from the grill and place them on serving plates.

7. Drizzle any remaining lemon-herb mixture over the top before serving.

Nutritional Values (per serving):

- Calories: 180

- Protein: 28g

- Carbohydrates: 5g

- Dietary Fiber: 2g

Cooking Tip: Grilling fish over high heat helps to seal in its natural juices. The fresh lemon and herbs complement the mild flavor of tilapia, making it a light and refreshing meal option.

Recipe 30: Stuffed Acorn Squash with Quinoa, Cranberries, and Spinach

Prep Time: 20 minutes - Cooking Time: 50 minutes - Number of Servings: 4

Ingredients:
- 2 medium acorn squashes halved, and seeds removed.
- 1 cup quinoa rinsed and drained.
- 2 cups vegetable broth
- 1 cup fresh spinach, chopped.
- 1/2 cup dried cranberries
- 1/4 cup walnuts, chopped (optional)
- 1 small onion finely diced.
- 2 garlic cloves, minced.
- 1 tsp olive oil or avocado oil
- Salt and pepper to taste.

Instructions:
1. Preheat your oven to 375°F (190°C).
2. Place the acorn squash halves, cut side down, on a baking sheet. Bake for about 30-35 minutes or until the squash is tender.
3. In a medium saucepan, bring the vegetable broth to a boil. Add the quinoa, reduce the heat to low, cover, and cook for 15 minutes, or until the quinoa is cooked and the liquid is absorbed. Remove from heat and set aside.
4. In a skillet, heat the olive oil or avocado oil over medium heat. Add the onion and sauté until translucent, about 4 minutes. Add the garlic and cook for another minute.
5. Stir in the chopped spinach and cook until wilted, about 2-3 minutes.
6. Remove from heat and add the cooked quinoa, dried cranberries, and chopped walnuts if using. Season with salt and pepper to taste.
7. Stuff each acorn squash in half with the quinoa mixture, pressing down slightly to pack the filling.
8. Return the stuffed squash halves to the oven and bake for an additional 10-15 minutes or until heated through.
9. Serve warm.

Nutritional Values (per serving):
- Calories: 320
- Protein: 8g
- Carbohydrates: 65g
- Dietary Fiber: 7g

Cooking Tip: Acorn squash is naturally sweet, and its flavor pairs wonderfully with the nuttiness of quinoa and tartness of cranberries.

Recipe 31: Chickpea and Vegetable Curry over Brown Rice

Prep Time: 20 minutes - Cooking Time: 30 minutes - Number of Servings: 4

Ingredients:

- 2 cups cooked brown rice
- 2 cans (14.5 oz each) of chickpeas rinsed and drained.
- 1 can (14.5 oz) diced tomatoes, undrained.
- 1 large carrot, diced.
- 1 bell pepper (any color), diced.
- 1 medium onion finely diced.
- 3 garlic cloves, minced.
- 2 tsp curry powder
- 1 tsp ground turmeric
- 1 tsp ground cumin
- 1/2 tsp chili powder (adjust for heat preference)
- 1 can (14 oz) light coconut milk
- Salt and pepper to taste.
- 1 tbsp olive oil or avocado oil
- Fresh cilantro, chopped (for garnish)

Instructions:

1. In a large pot or skillet, heat the olive oil or avocado oil over medium heat. Add the onion and sauté until translucent, about 4 minutes.
2. Add the garlic, curry powder, turmeric, cumin, and chili powder. Continue to sauté for another 2 minutes until fragrant.
3. Stir in the diced tomatoes (with their juices), chickpeas, carrots, and bell pepper.
4. Pour in the coconut milk and mix well.
5. Bring the mixture to a boil, then reduce the heat to low. Cover and let simmer for 20-25 minutes, stirring occasionally.
6. Season the curry with salt and pepper to taste.
7. Serve the chickpea and vegetable curry over cooked brown rice and garnish with fresh chopped cilantro.

Nutritional Values (per serving):

- Calories: 450

- Protein: 14g

- Carbohydrates: 75g

- Dietary Fiber: 12g

Cooking Tip: For added flavor, you can include a stick of cinnamon and a couple of cardamom pods while simmering the curry. Remember to remove them before serving.

Recipe 32: Spaghetti Squash Primavera with Fresh Vegetable Medley

Prep Time: 20 minutes - Cooking Time: 45 minutes - Number of Servings: 4

Ingredients:

- 1 medium spaghetti squash halved, and seeds removed.
- 1 cup cherry tomatoes, halved.
- 1 bell pepper (any color), diced.
- 1 zucchini, diced.
- 1 carrot, julienned or thinly sliced.
- 3 garlic cloves, minced.
- 1/4 cup fresh basil, chopped.
- 1/4 cup fresh parsley, chopped.
- Salt and pepper to taste.
- 2 tbsp olive oil or avocado oil
- Grated Parmesan cheese or nutritional yeast (optional for garnish)

Instructions:

1. Preheat your oven to 400°F (200°C).

2. Place the spaghetti squash halves, cut side down, on a baking sheet. Bake in the preheated oven for about 40-45 minutes or until the squash is tender.

3. In a large skillet, heat the olive oil or avocado oil over medium heat. Add the garlic and sauté until fragrant, about 1-2 minutes.

4. Add the cherry tomatoes, bell pepper, zucchini, and carrot to the skillet. Cook for about 5-7 minutes or until the vegetables are tender.

5. Once the spaghetti squash is done baking, use a fork to scrape out the flesh into thin strands, adding them directly to the skillet with the vegetables.

6. Toss the spaghetti squash and vegetables together until well combined. Stir in the fresh basil and parsley, and season with salt and pepper to taste.

7. Serve warm, garnishing with grated Parmesan cheese or nutritional yeast if desired.

Nutritional Values (per serving):

- Calories: 190

- Protein: 4g

- Carbohydrates: 33g

- Dietary Fiber: 7g

Cooking Tip: Spaghetti squash is a fantastic low-carb substitute for traditional pasta. Its neutral flavor pairs well with a variety of sauces and toppings.

Recipe 33: Grilled Eggplant and Tomato Stacks with Basil Drizzle

Prep Time: 20 minutes - Cooking Time: 15 minutes - Number of Servings: 4

Ingredients:

- 2 medium eggplants, sliced into 1/2-inch rounds.
- 3 large tomatoes, sliced.
- 1/4 cup fresh basil leaves
- 2 garlic cloves
- 2 tbsp pine nuts or walnuts
- 2 tbsp grated Parmesan cheese or nutritional yeast
- 1/4 cup extra-virgin olive oil, plus more for brushing
- Salt and pepper to taste.

Instructions:

1. Preheat your grill or grill pan to medium-high heat.

2. Brush both sides of the eggplant slices lightly with olive oil and season with salt and pepper.

3. Grill the eggplant slices for about 3-4 minutes on each side or until they have grill marks and are tender. Remove from the grill and set aside.

4. In a food processor, combine the basil leaves, garlic, nuts, and Parmesan cheese or nutritional yeast. Pulse until finely chopped. With the processor running, slowly pour in the 1/4 cup of olive oil until a smooth sauce is formed. Season with salt and pepper to taste.

5. To assemble the stacks, place an eggplant slice on a plate, followed by a tomato slice. Repeat this layering, finishing with an eggplant slice on top. Drizzle the basil sauce over the stacks.

6. Serve immediately.

Nutritional Values (per serving):

- Calories: 210

- Protein: 5g

- Carbohydrates: 18g

- Dietary Fiber: 9g

Cooking Tip: These eggplant and tomato stacks can also be served cold as a refreshing summer appetizer or side dish.

Recipe 34: Lentil and Vegetable Shepherd's Pie Topped with Cauliflower Mash

Prep Time: 25 minutes - Cooking Time: 40 minutes - Number of Servings: 4

Ingredients:

- 1 cup green or brown lentils rinsed and drained.
- 1 large head cauliflower, broken into florets.
- 2 carrots, diced.
- 1 onion finely diced.
- 2 garlic cloves, minced.
- 2 cups vegetable broth
- 1/2 cup green peas, fresh or frozen
- 1 tsp dried thyme
- 1 tsp dried rosemary
- Salt and pepper to taste.
- 2 tbsp olive oil or avocado oil

Instructions:

1. Preheat your oven to 375°F (190°C).
2. In a large pot, bring the vegetable broth to a boil. Add the lentils, reduce the heat to low, cover, and simmer for about 20-25 minutes, or until lentils are tender but not mushy.
3. While the lentils are cooking, steam the cauliflower florets until they are soft, about 10 minutes. Once steamed, transfer the cauliflower to a food processor. Process until smooth, adding a little water or broth if needed to achieve the consistency of mashed potatoes. Season with salt and pepper.

4. In a skillet, heat the olive oil or avocado oil over medium heat. Add the onion and sauté until translucent, about 4 minutes. Add the garlic, carrots, thyme, and rosemary, and continue to cook until the carrots are tender, about 5 minutes.
5. Add the cooked lentils and green peas to the skillet, stirring to combine. Adjust the seasoning with salt and pepper.
6. Transfer the lentil and vegetable mixture to a baking dish. Spread the cauliflower mash over the top, smoothing it out with a spatula.
7. Bake in the preheated oven for 20 minutes or until the top starts to turn golden.
8. Remove from the oven and let sit for a few minutes before serving.

Nutritional Values (per serving):

- Calories: 340
- Protein: 18g
- Carbohydrates: 56g
- Dietary Fiber: 23g

Cooking Tip: For an added touch of flavor, mix a little grated cheese or nutritional yeast into the cauliflower mash before baking.

Recipe 35: Barley Risotto with Mushrooms and Green Peas

Prep Time: 15 minutes - Cooking Time: 50 minutes - Number of Servings: 4

Ingredients:

- 1 cup pearl barley rinsed and drained.
- 4 cups vegetable broth
- 2 cups mixed mushrooms (e.g., cremini, shiitake, portobello), sliced.
- 1 cup green peas, fresh or frozen
- 1 onion finely chopped.
- 2 garlic cloves, minced.
- 1/2 cup dry white wine (optional)
- 1/4 cup fresh parsley, chopped.
- 1/4 cup grated Parmesan cheese or nutritional yeast
- Salt and pepper to taste.
- 2 tbsp olive oil or avocado oil

Instructions:

1. In a large pot or deep skillet, heat the olive oil or avocado oil over medium heat. Add the onion and sauté until translucent, about 4 minutes.
2. Add the garlic and mushrooms and continue to sauté for another 5 minutes, or until the mushrooms release their moisture and become tender.
3. Stir in the barley and cook for 2 minutes, allowing it to toast slightly.
4. If using, pour in the white wine and allow it to reduce by half.
5. Gradually add the vegetable broth, one cup at a time, stirring occasionally. Wait until most of the liquid is absorbed before adding the next cup.
6. When the barley is nearly done (about 40 minutes in), stir in the green peas. Continue to cook until the peas are heated through and the barley is tender yet slightly firm in the center.
7. Remove from heat and stir in the parsley and grated Parmesan cheese or nutritional yeast. Season with salt and pepper to taste.
8. Serve the barley risotto warm, garnishing with additional parsley or cheese if desired.

Nutritional Values (per serving):

- Calories: 310

- Protein: 12g

- Carbohydrates: 52g

- Dietary Fiber: 11g

Cooking Tip: Barley risotto is a wonderful, heart-healthy alternative to traditional rice risotto. Its natural nuttiness pairs well with earthy mushrooms and sweet peas.

Recipe 36: Black Bean and Corn Stuffed Poblano Peppers

Prep Time: 20 minutes - Cooking Time: 35 minutes - Number of Servings: 4

Ingredients:

- 4 large poblano peppers
- 1 can (14.5 oz) black beans rinsed and drained.
- 1 cup corn kernels (fresh, frozen, or canned)
- 1 cup cooked brown rice.
- 1 tomato, diced.
- 1/2 cup red onion finely chopped.
- 1 garlic clove, minced.
- 1 tsp ground cumin
- 1 tsp chili powder
- 1/4 cup fresh cilantro, chopped.
- Salt and pepper to taste.
- 1 tbsp olive oil or avocado oil
- Optional toppings: salsa, avocado slices, low-fat sour cream

Instructions:

1. Preheat your oven to 375°F (190°C).
2. In a large skillet, heat the olive oil or avocado oil over medium heat. Add the red onion and sauté until translucent, about 4 minutes. Add the garlic and cook for an additional minute.
3. Stir in the black beans, corn, tomato, cumin, and chili powder. Cook for 5-7 minutes until heated through. Add the cooked brown rice and mix well. Season with salt and pepper.
4. Remove from heat and stir in the fresh cilantro.
5. Make a slit in each poblano pepper from the stem to the tip. Gently open each pepper and remove the seeds and membranes.
6. Stuff each pepper with the black bean and corn mixture, pressing down gently to pack the filling.
7. Place the stuffed peppers in a baking dish and cover with aluminum foil.
8. Bake in the preheated oven for about 25-30 minutes or until the peppers are tender.
9. Serve warm with optional toppings if desired.

Nutritional Values (per serving):

- Calories: 270

- Protein: 10g

- Carbohydrates: 49g

- Dietary Fiber: 10g

Cooking Tip: If you like your dishes spicy, consider adding a diced jalapeño pepper to the black bean and corn mixture.

Recipe 37: Steamed Cod with Ginger and Scallion Sauce

Prep Time: 15 minutes - Cooking Time: 10 minutes - Number of Servings: 4

Ingredients:

- 4 cod fillets (about 56 oz each)
- 4 scallions thinly sliced.
- 2-inch piece of ginger peeled and julienned.
- 2 tbsp low sodium soy sauce or tamari
- 1 tbsp rice vinegar
- 1 tsp sesame oil
- 1/4 cup cilantro leaves, for garnish
- Olive oil or avocado oil spray

Instructions:

1. Prepare your steamer. If you don't have a dedicated steamer, you can set a heatproof dish on a rack inside a large skillet. Fill the skillet with enough water to come just below the rack. Bring the water to a boil.

2. Lightly spray the cod fillets with olive or avocado oil and place them in the steamer or on the heatproof dish. Cover and steam for about 7-10 minutes, depending on thickness, or until the fish flakes easily with a fork.

3. While the fish is steaming, in a small saucepan, combine the soy sauce, rice vinegar, and sesame oil. Heat over medium heat until it starts to simmer.

4. Add the julienned ginger to the saucepan and cook for about 1-2 minutes.

5. Once the fish is done, carefully transfer the fillets to serving plates.

6. Spoon the ginger and scallion sauce over the steamed cod fillets, garnish with cilantro leaves, and serve immediately.

Nutritional Values (per serving):

- Calories: 140

- Protein: 25g

- Carbohydrates: 2g

- Dietary Fiber: 0g

Cooking Tip: This dish is all about fresh and clean flavors. The ginger and scallion sauce provides a lovely, aromatic, and flavorful complement to the delicate taste of the cod.

Recipe 38: Turmeric and Vegetable Couscous with Roasted Chickpeas

Prep Time: 15 minutes - Cooking Time: 25 minutes - Number of Servings: 4

Ingredients:
- 1 cup couscous
- 1 1/4 cups vegetable broth
- 1 can (14.5 oz) chickpeas, rinsed, drained, and patted dry.
- 2 tbsp olive oil or avocado oil divided
- 1 tsp ground turmeric
- 1/2 tsp smoked paprika.
- 1 small zucchini, diced.
- 1 red bell pepper, diced.
- 1 carrot, diced.
- 1/4 cup fresh parsley, chopped.
- Salt and pepper to taste.

Instructions:
1. Preheat your oven to 400°F (200°C).
2. In a bowl, toss the chickpeas with 1 tbsp of olive or avocado oil, turmeric, smoked paprika, salt, and pepper. Spread them out on a baking sheet in a single layer.
3. Roast the chickpeas in the preheated oven for 20-25 minutes or until they're golden and slightly crispy. Shake the pan or stir the chickpeas halfway through to ensure even roasting.
4. While the chickpeas are roasting, heat the remaining 1 tbsp of oil in a large skillet over medium heat. Add the zucchini, bell pepper, and carrot. Sauté for about 5-7 minutes or until the vegetables are tender.
5. In a separate pot, bring the vegetable broth to a boil. Stir in the couscous, cover, and remove from heat. Let it stand for 5 minutes, then fluff it with a fork.
6. Combine the cooked couscous with the sautéed vegetables, and gently mix in the roasted chickpeas and fresh parsley.
7. Season with additional salt and pepper if needed and serve warm.

Nutritional Values (per serving):

- Calories: 300

- Protein: 9g

- Carbohydrates: 50g

- Dietary Fiber: 7g

Cooking Tip: Couscous is a quick-cooking grain, making it perfect for weeknight dinners. The turmeric not only adds flavor but also gives a lovely golden hue to the dish.

Recipe 39: Seared Tofu Steaks with Broccoli and Peanut Sauce (low-fat version)

Prep Time: 20 minutes - Cooking Time: 15 minutes - Number of Servings: 4

Ingredients:

- 1 block (14 oz) firm tofu, pressed and sliced into 1/2-inch thick steaks.
- 4 cups broccoli florets
- 2 garlic cloves, minced.
- 1-inch piece of ginger, grated.
- 3 tbsp low-sodium soy sauce or tamari
- 2 tbsp creamy peanut butter (natural, unsweetened)
- 1 tbsp rice vinegar
- 1 tsp maple syrup or honey
- 1 tsp chili flakes (adjust to taste)
- 1/4 cup warm water
- 2 tbsp olive oil or avocado oil
- Fresh cilantro for garnish
- Crushed peanuts for garnish (optional)

Instructions:

1. In a bowl, whisk together the minced garlic, grated ginger, soy sauce, peanut butter, rice vinegar, maple syrup, chili flakes, and warm water until smooth. Set the peanut sauce aside.

2. In a large skillet or wok, heat 1 tbsp of olive or avocado oil over medium-high heat. Add the tofu steaks and sear for about 3-4 minutes on each side or until they have a golden crust. Remove the tofu from the skillet and set aside.

3. In the same skillet, add the remaining 1 tbsp of oil. Sauté the broccoli florets for about 5-7 minutes or until they are tender-crisp.

4. Return the seared tofu to the skillet and pour the peanut sauce over the tofu and broccoli. Toss gently to coat everything in the sauce.

5. Continue to cook for another 2-3 minutes or until everything is heated through.

6. Serve the tofu and broccoli hot, garnished with fresh cilantro and crushed peanuts if desired.

Nutritional Values (per serving):

- Calories: 230
- Protein: 16g
- Carbohydrates: 16g
- Dietary Fiber: 4g

Cooking Tip: Pressing the tofu is crucial as it removes excess water, allowing the tofu to achieve a firmer texture when cooked. Using a tofu press or placing the tofu between two plates with a weight on top for about 15 minutes should do the trick.

Recipe 40: Vegetable Paella with Saffron and Artichokes

Prep Time: 20 minutes - Cooking Time: 40 minutes - Number of Servings: 4

Ingredients:

- 1 1/2 cups Arborio rice
- 3 1/2 cups vegetable broth
- 1/2 cup dry white wine (optional)
- 1 red bell pepper, diced
- 1 yellow bell pepper, diced
- 1 onion, finely chopped
- 2 cloves garlic, minced
- 1 cup frozen green peas
- 1 can (14 oz) artichoke hearts, drained and quartered
- 1 tsp saffron threads (soaked in 2 tbsp warm water)
- 1 tsp smoked paprika
- 1/2 tsp ground turmeric
- 1/2 tsp cayenne pepper (adjust to taste)
- 1/4 cup fresh parsley, chopped
- Olive oil or avocado oil for sautéing
- Lemon wedges, for garnish

Instructions:

1. In a large skillet or paella pan, heat a bit of olive oil or avocado oil over medium heat. Add the diced onion and bell peppers. Sauté for about 5 minutes or until they start to soften.

2. Add the minced garlic and sauté for an additional minute until fragrant.

3. Stir in the Arborio rice, smoked paprika, ground turmeric, and cayenne pepper. Cook for 2-3 minutes, allowing the rice to toast slightly.

4. If using white wine, pour it into the skillet and stir until mostly absorbed by the rice.

5. Pour in the vegetable broth, saffron threads with their soaking water, and a pinch of salt. Bring to a gentle boil, then reduce the heat to low. Cover and simmer for about 20-25 minutes or until the rice is tender and has absorbed the liquid.

6. About 5 minutes before the rice is done, gently fold in the frozen green peas and artichoke hearts.

7. Taste and adjust the seasoning with salt and pepper if needed.

8. Garnish the vegetable paella with fresh chopped parsley and serve hot with lemon wedges for squeezing over the top.

Nutritional Values (per serving):

- Calories: 370
- Protein: 7g
- Carbohydrates: 74g
- Dietary Fiber: 6g

Recipe 41: Lemon-Pepper Roasted Brussels Sprouts and Tempeh Bowl

Prep Time: 15 minutes - Cooking Time: 30 minutes - Number of Servings: 4

Ingredients:

- 1 cup dry quinoa
- 2 cups water
- 8 oz tempeh, cut into cubes.
- 1 lb. Brussels sprouts trimmed and halved.
- 2 lemons zested and juiced.
- 2 tbsp olive oil or avocado oil
- 2 tsp ground black pepper
- 1 tsp garlic powder
- 1/4 cup fresh parsley, chopped.
- Salt to taste
- Lemon wedges, for garnish

Instructions:

1. Preheat your oven to 400°F (200°C).
2. In a saucepan, combine the quinoa and water. Bring to a boil, then reduce the heat to low, cover, and simmer for about 15-20 minutes, or until the quinoa is cooked and the water is absorbed.
3. While the quinoa is cooking, in a mixing bowl, combine the cubed tempeh, Brussels sprouts, lemon zest, lemon juice, olive oil, black pepper, garlic powder, and a pinch of salt. Toss until everything is evenly coated.
4. Spread the tempeh and Brussels sprouts mixture on a baking sheet in a single layer.
5. Roast in the preheated oven for 20-25 minutes or until the Brussels sprouts are tender and caramelized and the tempeh is crispy.
6. Fluff the cooked quinoa with a fork and divide it among serving bowls.
7. Top the quinoa with the lemon-pepper roasted Brussels sprouts and tempeh.
8. Garnish with freshly chopped parsley and lemon wedges for an extra burst of flavor.

Nutritional Values (per serving):

- Calories: 370

- Protein: 21g

- Carbohydrates: 43g

- Dietary Fiber: 8g

Cooking Tip: Roasting tempeh with Brussels sprouts not only adds a delightful crunch but also infuses the dish with a zesty lemon-pepper flavor.

Recipe 42: Moroccan Vegetable and Chickpea Tagine

Prep Time: 20 minutes - Cooking Time: 45 minutes - Number of Servings: 4

Ingredients:

- 2 tbsp olive oil or avocado oil
- 1 onion finely chopped.
- 2 garlic cloves, minced.
- 1 tsp ground cumin
- 1 tsp ground coriander
- 1 tsp ground cinnamon
- 1/2 tsp ground ginger
- 1/2 tsp ground paprika
- 1/4 tsp cayenne pepper (adjust to taste)
- 1 can (14.5 oz) diced tomatoes.
- 1 can (14.5 oz) chickpeas rinsed and drained.
- 2 carrots peeled and diced.
- 1 sweet potato peeled and diced.
- 1 red bell pepper, diced.
- 1 zucchini, diced.
- 1 cup vegetable broth
- 1/4 cup dried apricots, chopped.
- 1/4 cup slivered almonds, toasted.
- Fresh cilantro leaves for garnish
- Salt and pepper to taste.
- Cooked couscous or quinoa for serving (optional)

Instructions:

1. In a large, deep skillet or tagine (if available), heat the olive oil or avocado oil over medium heat. Add the chopped onion and sauté for about 3-4 minutes until it begins to soften.

2. Stir in the minced garlic and cook for an additional minute until fragrant.

3. Add the ground cumin, coriander, cinnamon, ginger, paprika, and cayenne pepper to the skillet. Stir well to coat the onions and garlic with the spices.

4. Pour in the diced tomatoes and their juice, chickpeas, carrots, sweet potato, red bell pepper, and zucchini.

5. Add the vegetable broth, dried apricots, and a pinch of salt and pepper. Stir to combine.

6. Cover and simmer over low heat for about 30-35 minutes, or until the vegetables are tender and the flavors have melded together.

7. While the tagine is cooking, toast the slivered almonds in a dry skillet over medium-low heat until they turn golden, about 3-4 minutes. Keep a close eye on them, as they can burn quickly.

8. Serve the Moroccan vegetable and chickpea tagine hot, garnished with toasted slivered almonds and fresh cilantro leaves. You can also serve it over cooked couscous or quinoa if desired.

Nutritional Values (per serving):

- Calories: 350
- Protein: 10g
- Carbohydrates: 59g
- Dietary Fiber: 14g

Cooking Tip: Tagine dishes are often cooked in a special clay pot called a tagine, but a deep skillet with a lid works well as a substitute.

Chapter 9: Sides Recipes

Welcome to Chapter 9 of "*Pritikin Diet For Seniors: The Complete Guide to Weight Loss and Improved Health for Seniors.*" Side dishes play a role in creating a balanced and satisfying meal. In this chapter, we are excited to present a collection of side dish recipes that will enhance your dining experience and align with your wellness goals.

Our crafted side dish recipes offer an array of nutritious options that perfectly complement your main courses. These dishes aim to bring variety to your meals while helping you maintain weight.

From salads to vegetable preparations, these recipes showcase the versatility and deliciousness of plant-based ingredients. We have incorporated an array of herbs, spices, and seasonings to create side dishes that are both tempting and nourishing.

At Pritikin, we strongly believe in the power of ingredients, and these side dish recipes reflect that philosophy. You will find options that are not only delicious but also mindful of your journey toward longevity and well-being.

So, as you explore the recipes in this chapter, you will discover that side dishes can be more than accompaniments: they can take the stage on your plate.

These side dish recipes will bring a burst of flavor and nutrition to your meals, helping you reach your weight management goals and improve your health with each delicious bite.

Chapter 9: Pritikin Sides Delights

43. Garlic Steamed Green Beans with Toasted Almonds

44. Roasted Root Vegetables with Fresh Rosemary

45. Cilantro-Lime Brown Rice Pilaf

46. Sautéed Kale with Golden Raisins and Pine Nuts (minimal oil)

47. Grilled Asparagus Spears with Lemon Zest

48. Mashed Butternut Squash with a Hint of Nutmeg

49. Fresh Tomato, Cucumber, and Red Onion Salad

50. Broccoli and Cauliflower Florets with Tahini Drizzle

51. Warm Beet Salad with Orange Segments

52. Brussel Sprouts with Balsamic Reduction and Cranberries

53. Sweet Corn and Edamame Succotash

54. Baked Spinach and Artichoke Dip (low-fat version)

55. Quinoa and Black Bean Salad with Mango and Avocado

56. Roasted Red Pepper and Walnut Spread (low-fat version)

These side dish recipes emphasize the natural flavors and textures of fresh produce and grains, complementing the main courses and adhering to the principles of the Pritikin Diet.

Recipe 43: Garlic Steamed Green Beans with Toasted Almonds

Prep Time: 10 minutes - Cooking Time: 10 minutes - Number of Servings: 4

Ingredients:

- 1 lb. fresh green beans, trimmed.
- 2 cloves garlic, minced.
- 1/4 cup sliced almonds, toasted.
- 1 tbsp olive oil or avocado oil
- Salt and pepper to taste.
- Lemon wedges, for garnish (optional)

Instructions:

1. In a large pot, bring about 1 inch of water to a boil. Add a steamer basket to the pot.

2. Place the green beans in the steamer basket, cover, and steam for about 5-7 minutes, or until they are tender yet still crisp.

3. While the green beans are steaming, heat the olive oil or avocado oil in a skillet over medium heat. Add the minced garlic and sauté for about 1 minute, or until fragrant but not browned.

4. Remove the green beans from the steamer basket and transfer them to a serving platter.

5. Drizzle the garlic-infused oil over the green beans. Sprinkle with toasted sliced almonds.

6. Season with salt and pepper to taste and garnish with lemon wedges if desired.

Nutritional Values (per serving):

- Calories: 90

- Protein: 3g

- Carbohydrates: 8g

- Dietary Fiber: 4g

Cooking Tip: Steaming the green beans preserves their vibrant color and crisp texture. The toasted almonds add a delightful crunch and nutty flavor to this simple side dish.

Recipe 44: Roasted Root Vegetables with Fresh Rosemary

Prep Time: 15 minutes - Cooking Time: 35 minutes - Number of Servings: 4

Ingredients:

- 4 cups mixed root vegetables (e.g., carrots, parsnips, sweet potatoes, beets), peeled and cut into 1-inch pieces.
- 2 tbsp olive oil or avocado oil
- 2 sprigs fresh rosemary, leaves stripped and chopped.
- Salt and pepper to taste.

Instructions:

1. Preheat your oven to 425°F (220°C).

2. In a large mixing bowl, combine the root vegetables with the olive oil, chopped fresh rosemary, salt, and pepper. Toss until the vegetables are evenly coated.

3. Spread the seasoned vegetables in a single layer on a baking sheet.

4. Roast in the preheated oven for about 30-35 minutes, or until the vegetables are tender and caramelized, stirring once or twice during cooking for even browning.

5. Serve the roasted root vegetables hot.

Nutritional Values (per serving):

- Calories: 160
- Protein: 2g
- Carbohydrates: 24g
- Dietary Fiber: 6g

Cooking Tip: Roasting root vegetables brings out their natural sweetness and creates a deliciously crispy exterior. Fresh rosemary adds a fragrant and earthy note to this dish.

Recipe 45: Cilantro-Lime Brown Rice Pilaf

Prep Time: 10 minutes - Cooking Time: 40 minutes - Number of Servings: 4

Ingredients:

- 1 cup brown rice
- 2 cups vegetable broth
- 1 lime, zest, and juice
- 1/2 cup fresh cilantro leaves, chopped.
- 1/4 cup red onion finely chopped.
- 1 clove garlic, minced.
- 1 tbsp olive oil or avocado oil
- Salt and pepper to taste.
- Lime wedges for garnish (optional)

Instructions:

1. Rinse the brown rice under cold running water until the water runs clear.

2. In a medium saucepan, heat the olive oil or avocado oil over medium heat. Add the minced garlic and chopped red onion. Sauté for about 2-3 minutes or until they begin to soften.

3. Stir in the rinsed brown rice and sauté for an additional 2 minutes, allowing the rice to lightly toast.

4. Pour in the vegetable broth and bring to a boil. Reduce the heat to low, cover, and simmer for about 35-40 minutes, or until the rice is tender and has absorbed all the liquid.

5. Fluff the cooked rice with a fork, then stir in the lime zest, lime juice, and fresh chopped cilantro. Season with salt and pepper to taste.

6. Serve the cilantro-lime brown rice pilaf hot, garnished with lime wedges if desired.

Nutritional Values (per serving):

- Calories: 180

- Protein: 3g

- Carbohydrates: 35g

- Dietary Fiber: 2g

Cooking Tip: The combination of fresh cilantro and zesty lime gives this brown rice pilaf a burst of new flavor. It's a perfect side dish for a variety of main courses.

Recipe 46: Sautéed Kale with Golden Raisins and Pine Nuts (minimal oil)

Prep Time: 10 minutes - Cooking Time: 10 minutes - Number of Servings: 4

Ingredients:

- 1 bunch kale, stems removed, and leaves chopped.
- 2 tbsp pine nuts
- 2 tbsp golden raisins
- 1 clove garlic, minced.
- 1 tbsp olive oil or avocado oil
- Salt and pepper to taste.
- Lemon wedges, for garnish (optional)

Instructions:

1. In a large skillet, toast the pine nuts over medium-low heat for about 2-3 minutes or until they turn golden. Be attentive, as they can burn quickly. Remove them from the skillet and set aside.

2. In the same skillet, heat the olive oil or avocado oil over medium heat. Add the minced garlic and sauté for about 30 seconds or until fragrant.

3. Add the chopped kale and stir-fry for about 3-4 minutes, or until the kale has wilted and is tender-crisp.

4. Stir in the golden raisins and toasted pine nuts. Continue to cook for an additional 2 minutes or until the raisins plump up slightly.

5. Season with salt and pepper to taste.

6. Serve the sautéed kale hot, garnished with lemon wedges if desired.

Nutritional Values (per serving):

- Calories: 120

- Protein: 3g

- Carbohydrates: 14g

- Dietary Fiber: 2g

Cooking Tip: Sautéing kale with a touch of oil and adding sweet golden raisins and crunchy pine nuts creates a delightful combination of flavors and textures.

Recipe 47: Grilled Asparagus Spears with Lemon Zest

Prep Time: 10 minutes - Cooking Time: 10 minutes - Number of Servings: 4

Ingredients:

- 1 lb. fresh asparagus spears, tough ends trimmed.
- 1 lemon, zest, and juice
- 1 tbsp olive oil or avocado oil
- Salt and pepper to taste.

Instructions:

1. Preheat your grill to medium-high heat.

2. In a bowl, combine the fresh asparagus spears, olive oil, and a pinch of salt and pepper. Toss to coat the asparagus evenly.

3. Place the asparagus spears on the grill and cook for about 4-5 minutes per side or until they are tender and have grill marks.

4. While the asparagus is grilling, zest the lemon and set the zest aside.

5. Remove the grilled asparagus from the grill and transfer it to a serving platter.

6. Drizzle the lemon juice over the asparagus and sprinkle with lemon zest.

7. Season with additional salt and pepper if needed.

Nutritional Values (per serving):

- Calories: 40

- Protein: 2g

- Carbohydrates: 4g

- Dietary Fiber: 2g

Cooking Tip: Grilling asparagus enhances its natural flavor and adds a delightful smokiness. The lemon zest and juice provide a refreshing and zesty finish.

Recipe 48: Mashed Butternut Squash with a Hint of Nutmeg

Prep Time: 15 minutes - Cooking Time: 25 minutes - Number of Servings: 4

Ingredients:

- 1 medium butternut squash, peeled, seeded, and cut into chunks.
- 1/4 cup unsweetened almond milk or vegetable broth
- 1/2 tsp ground nutmeg
- 1/4 tsp ground cinnamon
- Salt and pepper to taste.
- Fresh chives for garnish (optional)

Instructions:

1. Place the butternut squash chunks in a large pot of boiling water. Cook for about 15-20 minutes or until the squash is fork-tender.

2. Drain the cooked squash and transfer it to a mixing bowl.

3. Use a potato masher or a hand blender to mash the butternut squash until smooth.

4. Stir in the almond milk or vegetable broth, ground nutmeg, ground cinnamon, salt, and pepper. Continue to mash and mix until you achieve your desired consistency.

5. Taste and adjust the seasonings if needed.

6. Serve the mashed butternut squash hot, garnished with fresh chives if desired.

Nutritional Values (per serving):

- Calories: 70

- Protein: 2g

- Carbohydrates: 18g

- Dietary Fiber: 4g

Cooking Tip: The addition of nutmeg and cinnamon brings warmth and depth to this mashed butternut squash dish, making it a comforting and nutritious side.

Recipe 49: Fresh Tomato, Cucumber, and Red Onion Salad

Prep Time: 10 minutes - Cooking Time: 0 minutes - Number of Servings: 4

Ingredients:

- 4 ripe tomatoes, diced.
- 1 cucumber, diced.
- 1/2 red onion thinly sliced.
- 2 tbsp fresh parsley, chopped.
- 2 tbsp fresh mint, chopped.
- 2 tbsp extra virgin olive oil
- 1 tbsp red wine vinegar
- Salt and pepper to taste.

Instructions:

1. In a large bowl, combine the diced tomatoes, diced cucumber, thinly sliced red onion, chopped fresh parsley, and chopped fresh mint.

2. In a small bowl, whisk together the extra-virgin olive oil and red wine vinegar.

3. Drizzle the dressing over the salad and toss to coat all the ingredients.

4. Season with salt and pepper to taste.

5. Let the salad sit for a few minutes to allow the flavors to meld before serving.

Nutritional Values (per serving):

- Calories: 90

- Protein: 2g

- Carbohydrates: 9g

- Dietary Fiber: 2g

Cooking Tip: This refreshing tomato, cucumber, and red onion salad is perfect for a light and healthy side dish. The combination of fresh herbs and a simple vinaigrette enhances the natural flavors of the ingredients.

Recipe 50: Broccoli and Cauliflower Florets with Tahini Drizzle

Prep Time: 10 minutes - Cooking Time: 10 minutes - Number of Servings: 4

Ingredients:

- 2 cups broccoli florets
- 2 cups cauliflower florets
- 2 tbsp tahini
- 1 lemon, juiced.
- 1 clove garlic, minced.
- 2 tbsp water
- Salt and pepper to taste.
- Sesame seeds and chopped fresh parsley, for garnish (optional)

Instructions:

1. In a pot of boiling water, blanch the broccoli and cauliflower florets for about 2-3 minutes until they are bright green and slightly tender. Drain and set aside.

2. In a small bowl, whisk together the tahini, lemon juice, minced garlic, and water to create a creamy dressing. Add more water if needed to reach your desired consistency.

3. Drizzle the tahini dressing over the blanched broccoli and cauliflower florets.

4. Season with salt and pepper to taste.

5. Garnish with sesame seeds and chopped fresh parsley if desired.

6. Serve the broccoli and cauliflower florets with tahini drizzle immediately.

Nutritional Values (per serving):

- Calories: 80

- Protein: 3g

- Carbohydrates: 8g

- Dietary Fiber: 3g

Cooking Tip: Tahini adds a rich and nutty flavor to the steamed broccoli and cauliflower, while the lemon juice provides a zesty contrast.

Recipe 51: Warm Beet Salad with Orange Segments

Prep Time: 15 minutes - Cooking Time: 45 minutes (for roasting beets) - Number of Servings: 4

Ingredients:

- 4 medium beets scrubbed and trimmed.
- 2 oranges, segmented.
- 1/4 cup red onion thinly sliced.
- 1/4 cup fresh mint leaves, chopped.
- 2 tbsp extra virgin olive oil
- 1 tbsp red wine vinegar
- Salt and pepper to taste.

Instructions:

1. Preheat your oven to 400°F (200°C).

2. Wrap each beet individually in aluminum foil and place them on a baking sheet.

3. Roast the beets in the preheated oven for about 45 minutes or until they are tender when pierced with a fork.

4. Remove the beets from the oven, let them cool, and then peel and dice them.

5. In a large bowl, combine the diced roasted beets, orange segments, thinly sliced red onion, and chopped fresh mint.

6. In a small bowl, whisk together the extra-virgin olive oil and red wine vinegar to create a simple vinaigrette.

7. Drizzle the vinaigrette over the salad and toss gently to combine.

8. Season with salt and pepper to taste.

9. Serve the warm beet salad immediately.

Nutritional Values (per serving):

- Calories: 120

- Protein: 2g

- Carbohydrates: 17g

- Dietary Fiber: 5g

Cooking Tip: Roasting beets intensifies their natural sweetness and earthy flavor. The combination of beets, oranges, and fresh mint creates a vibrant and refreshing salad.

Recipe 52: Brussel Sprouts with Balsamic Reduction and Cranberries

Prep Time: 10 minutes - Cooking Time: 20 minutes - Number of Servings: 4

Ingredients:

- 1 lb. Brussels sprouts trimmed and halved.
- 1/2 cup dried cranberries
- 2 tbsp balsamic vinegar
- 1 tbsp olive oil or avocado oil
- Salt and pepper to taste.
- 1/4 cup chopped pecans, toasted (optional)

Instructions:

1. Preheat your oven to 400°F (200°C).

2. In a large bowl, combine the Brussels sprouts, dried cranberries, olive oil, balsamic vinegar, salt, and pepper. Toss until the Brussels sprouts are evenly coated.

3. Spread the mixture on a baking sheet in a single layer.

4. Roast in the preheated oven for about 15-20 minutes, or until the Brussels sprouts are tender and caramelized, stirring once or twice during cooking for even browning.

5. If desired, toast the chopped pecans in a dry skillet over medium-low heat until they turn golden, about 3-4 minutes. Keep a close eye on them, as they can burn quickly.

6. Serve the roasted Brussels sprouts and cranberries hot, garnished with toasted pecans if desired.

Nutritional Values (per serving):

- Calories: 160

- Protein: 3g

- Carbohydrates: 28g

- Dietary Fiber: 5g

Cooking Tip: The sweet-tart combination of balsamic reduction and dried cranberries complements the earthy flavor of roasted Brussels sprouts. Toasted pecans add an extra layer of crunch and nuttiness.

Recipe 53: Sweet Corn and Edamame Succotash

Prep Time: 10 minutes - Cooking Time: 15 minutes - Number of Servings: 4

Ingredients:

- 2 cups fresh or frozen sweet corn kernels
- 1 cup shelled edamame (green soybeans)
- 1 red bell pepper, diced.
- 1/2 red onion finely chopped.
- 2 cloves garlic, minced.
- 2 tbsp olive oil or avocado oil
- 2 tbsp fresh basil, chopped.
- Salt and pepper to taste.
- Fresh lime wedges, for garnish (optional)

Instructions:

1. In a large skillet, heat the olive oil or avocado oil over medium heat.

2. Add the minced garlic and sauté for about 30 seconds or until fragrant.

3. Stir in the diced red onion and sauté for 2-3 minutes, or until it begins to soften.

4. Add the diced red bell pepper and continue to sauté for another 2-3 minutes until the pepper is tender.

5. Stir in the sweet corn kernels and shelled edamame. Cook for about 5-7 minutes or until the vegetables are heated through and slightly tender.

6. Season the succotash with salt and pepper to taste.

7. Remove from heat and stir in the fresh chopped basil.

8. Serve the sweet corn and edamame succotash hot, garnished with fresh lime wedges if desired.

Nutritional Values (per serving):

- Calories: 180

- Protein: 8g

- Carbohydrates: 26g

- Dietary Fiber: 5g

Cooking Tip: Succotash is a colorful and nutritious dish that celebrates the flavors of fresh summer vegetables. It's a perfect site for a variety of main courses.

Recipe 54: Baked Spinach and Artichoke Dip (low-fat version)

Prep Time: 15 minutes - Cooking Time: 25 minutes - Number of Servings: 4

Ingredients:

- 1 (10 oz) package of frozen chopped spinach, thawed and drained
- 1 (14 oz) can artichoke hearts, drained and chopped
- 1 cup low-fat Greek yogurt
- 1/2 cup grated Parmesan cheese
- 1/2 cup shredded part-skim mozzarella cheese
- 1/4 cup chopped green onions.
- 1 clove garlic, minced.
- 1/2 tsp red pepper flakes (optional)
- Salt and pepper to taste.
- Whole grain pita chips or fresh vegetable sticks for serving.

Instructions:

1. Preheat your oven to 350°F (175°C).

2. In a large mixing bowl, combine the thawed and drained chopped spinach, chopped artichoke hearts, low-fat Greek yogurt, grated Parmesan cheese, shredded mozzarella cheese, chopped green onions, minced garlic, and red pepper flakes (if using). Mix until all ingredients are well combined.

3. Season the mixture with salt and pepper to taste.

4. Transfer the mixture to a baking dish and spread it evenly.

5. Bake in the preheated oven for about 20-25 minutes, or until the dip is hot and bubbly and the top is lightly golden.

6. Remove from the oven and let it cool for a few minutes before serving.

7. Serve the baked spinach and artichoke dip with whole-grain pita chips or fresh vegetable sticks.

Nutritional Values (per serving, without chips or vegetable sticks):

- Calories: 150

- Protein: 12g

- Carbohydrates: 10g

- Dietary Fiber: 3g

Cooking Tip: This lighter version of spinach and artichoke dip uses Greek yogurt instead of sour cream and mayonnaise, making it a healthier option for dipping.

Recipe 55: Quinoa and Black Bean Salad with Mango and Avocado

Prep Time: 15 minutes - Cooking Time: 15 minutes - Number of Servings: 4

Ingredients:

- 1 cup quinoa rinsed and drained.
- 2 cups water or vegetable broth
- 1 mango, peeled, pitted, and diced.
- 1 avocado, peeled, pitted, and diced.
- 1 (15 oz) can black beans, drained and rinsed
- 1/2 red onion finely chopped.
- 1/4 cup fresh cilantro, chopped.
- Juice of 2 limes
- 2 tbsp extra-virgin olive oil
- Salt and pepper to taste.

Instructions:

1. In a medium saucepan, combine the quinoa and water or vegetable broth. Bring to a boil, then reduce the heat to low, cover, and simmer for about 15 minutes, or until the quinoa is cooked and the liquid is absorbed. Remove from heat and let it cool.

2. In a large mixing bowl, combine the cooked quinoa, diced mango, diced avocado, drained and rinsed black beans, finely chopped red onion, and chopped fresh cilantro.

3. In a small bowl, whisk together the lime juice and extra-virgin olive oil to create a zesty dressing.

4. Drizzle the dressing over the salad and toss to combine.

5. Season with salt and pepper to taste.

6. Serve the quinoa and black bean salad chilled.

Nutritional Values (per serving):

- Calories: 330

- Protein: 10g

- Carbohydrates: 48g

- Dietary Fiber: 11g

Cooking Tip: This vibrant salad combines the earthiness of quinoa and black beans with the sweetness of mango and the creaminess of avocado. It's a flavorful and satisfying side dish or light meal.

Recipe 56: Roasted Red Pepper and Walnut Spread (low-fat version)

Prep Time: 15 minutes - Cooking Time: 15 minutes - Number of Servings: 4

Ingredients:
- 2 large red bell peppers
- 1/2 cup walnuts, toasted.
- 1/4 cup low-fat plain Greek yogurt
- 2 cloves garlic, minced.
- 1 tsp lemon juice
- 1/2 tsp ground cumin
- 1/4 tsp smoked paprika.
- Salt and pepper to taste.
- Fresh parsley, for garnish (optional)

Instructions:
1. Preheat your broiler or grill to high heat.
2. Place the whole red bell peppers directly on the grill or under the broiler. Cook for about 5-7 minutes per side, turning occasionally, until the peppers are charred and blistered on all sides.
3. Remove the peppers from the grill or broiler and place them in a bowl. Cover the bowl with plastic wrap and let the peppers steam for about 10 minutes. This will make it easier to remove the skin.
4. After steaming, peel off the charred skin from the peppers, remove the seeds, and chop the flesh into smaller pieces.
5. In a food processor, combine the roasted red pepper pieces, toasted walnuts, low-fat plain Greek yogurt, minced garlic, lemon juice, ground cumin, and smoked paprika.
6. Pulse until the mixture reaches your desired consistency, scraping down the sides of the processor as needed.
7. Season the spread with salt and pepper to taste.
8. Serve the roasted red pepper and walnut spread garnished with fresh parsley if desired.

Nutritional Values (per serving):

- Calories: 130

- Protein: 4g

- Carbohydrates: 9g

- Dietary Fiber: 2g

Cooking Tip: Roasting red bell peppers adds a smoky flavor to this spread, while toasted walnuts provide a rich and nutty undertone. It's a delicious and healthy accompaniment for whole grain crackers or vegetable sticks.

Chapter 10: Dessert Recipes

Welcome to Chapter 10 of *"Pritikin Diet For Seniors: The Complete Guide to Weight Loss and Improved Health for Seniors,"* Desserts are the way to end a meal, and in this chapter, we invite you to indulge sensibly in a delightful variety of dessert recipes that align with your goals for health and longevity.

Our dessert recipes demonstrate that you can enjoy the side of life while still maintaining weight. We understand the importance of treats for a rounded lifestyle, and these recipes are carefully designed to help you satisfy your sweet cravings without compromising your health.

From guilty fruit-based desserts to lower-calorie versions of beloved classics, this chapter presents a diverse range of options to please every sweet tooth. Each recipe is crafted with ingredients and mindful portion control, ensuring that you can savor dessert with confidence.

As you explore these dessert recipes, you will discover that healthy eating does not mean giving up on the joys of indulgence. Instead, it's about making choices and relishing each bite while supporting your well-being and longevity.

Come along with us on an adventure as we delve into dessert recipes that demonstrate how you can indulge in your love for cake while still maintaining a lifestyle. These recipes will show you that enjoying dessert can be an enjoyable aspect of your Pritikin way of living. They will help you reach your weight management goals while allowing you to savor the joys of life.

Chapter 10: Pritikin Dessert Delights

57. Chilled Melon Balls with Fresh Mint and Lime Zest

58. Baked Apples Stuffed with Oats and Raisins

59. Berry and Kiwi Fruit Salad with a Lemon-Honey Drizzle

60. Cinnamon-Spiced Poached Pears

61. Mango and Chia Seed Pudding (no added sugars)

62. Dark Chocolate Dipped Strawberries (minimal chocolate)

63. Vanilla and Berry Frozen Yogurt Bark (low-fat version)

These dessert recipes aim to satisfy sweet cravings while staying true to the principles of the Pritikin Diet, emphasizing natural sweetness and minimal added fats or sugars.

Recipe 57: Chilled Melon Balls with Fresh Mint and Lime Zest

Prep Time: 15 minutes - Cooking Time: 0 minutes - Number of Servings: 4

Ingredients:

- 1 small cantaloupe melon, seeded and scooped into balls or cubes.
- 1 small honeydew melon, seeded and scooped into balls or cubes.
- Fresh mint leaves, for garnish
- Zest of 1 lime
- Lime wedges for garnish (optional)

Instructions:

1. In a large bowl, combine the cantaloupe and honeydew melon balls or cubes.

2. Sprinkle the fresh mint leaves over the melon.

3. Zest the lime directly over the melon to add a burst of citrusy flavor.

4. Gently toss the melon, mint, and lime zest together.

5. Chill the melon in the refrigerator for about 15 minutes before serving.

6. Optionally, garnish with lime wedges.

7. Serve the chilled melon balls immediately.

Nutritional Values (per serving):

- Calories: 60

- Protein: 1g

- Carbohydrates: 16g

- Dietary Fiber: 2g

Cooking Tip: This refreshing dessert combines the natural sweetness of melons with the zesty freshness of lime and the aromatic touch of mint.

Recipe 58: Baked Apples Stuffed with Oats and Raisins

Prep Time: 15 minutes - Cooking Time: 40 minutes - Number of Servings: 4

Ingredients:

- 4 medium apples (e.g., Granny Smith or Honeycrisp)
- 1/2 cup old-fashioned oats
- 1/4 cup raisins
- 1/4 cup chopped walnuts (optional)
- 2 tbsp honey or maple syrup (optional for added sweetness)
- 1 tsp ground cinnamon
- 1/2 tsp vanilla extract
- 1/2 cup water

Instructions:

1. Preheat your oven to 350°F (175°C).
2. Core the apples, creating a cavity in the center but leaving the base intact to form a cup.
3. In a bowl, combine the old-fashioned oats, raisins, chopped walnuts (if using), honey or maple syrup (if using), ground cinnamon, and vanilla extract. Mix until well combined.
4. Stuff each apple with the oat and raisin mixture, filling the cavity.
5. Place the stuffed apples in a baking dish.
6. Pour the water into the bottom of the dish to prevent the apples from sticking.
7. Cover the dish with aluminum foil and bake in the preheated oven for about 30-40 minutes or until the apples are tender.
8. Remove the foil for the last 10 minutes of baking to allow the tops to brown slightly.
9. Serve the baked apples hot, optionally drizzled with a little honey or maple syrup.

Nutritional Values (per serving, without honey/maple syrup or walnuts):

- Calories: 150

- Protein: 3g

- Carbohydrates: 36g

- Dietary Fiber: 6g

Cooking Tip: Baked apples stuffed with oats and raisins are a warm and comforting dessert. Adjust the sweetness to your liking with optional honey or maple syrup.

Recipe 59: Berry and Kiwi Fruit Salad with a Lemon-Honey Drizzle

Prep Time: 15 minutes - Cooking Time: 0 minutes - Number of Servings: 4

Ingredients:

- 2 cups mixed berries (e.g., strawberries, blueberries, raspberries)
- 2 kiwi fruits peeled and sliced.
- Zest and juice of 1 lemon
- 2 tbsp honey
- Fresh mint leaves, for garnish (optional)

Instructions:

1. In a large bowl, combine the mixed berries and sliced kiwi fruits.

2. In a small bowl, whisk together the lemon zest, lemon juice, and honey to create a drizzling sauce.

3. Drizzle the lemon-honey mixture over the fruit salad.

4. Gently toss to coat the fruit with the drizzle.

5. Optionally, garnish with fresh mint leaves.

6. Serve the berry and kiwi fruit salad immediately.

Nutritional Values (per serving):

- Calories: 90

- Protein: 1g

- Carbohydrates: 24g

- Dietary Fiber: 4g

Cooking Tip: This fruit salad combines the natural sweetness of berries and kiwi with a zesty lemon-honey drizzle for a light and delightful dessert.

Recipe 60: Cinnamon-Spiced Poached Pears

Prep Time: 10 minutes - Cooking Time: 30 minutes - Number of Servings: 4

Ingredients:

- 4 ripe but firm pears, peeled, halved, and cored.
- 2 cups water
- 1/2 cup apple juice (unsweetened)
- 1/4 cup honey or maple syrup
- 2 cinnamon sticks
- 1 tsp vanilla extract
- Zest of 1 orange
- 4 whole cloves (optional)

Instructions:

1. In a large saucepan, combine the water, apple juice, honey or maple syrup, cinnamon sticks, vanilla extract, orange zest, and whole cloves (if using). Bring the mixture to a boil.

2. Reduce the heat to low and add the pear halves to the poaching liquid.

3. Simmer gently for about 20-30 minutes or until the pears are tender when pierced with a fork. The exact time will depend on the ripeness of your pears.

4. Once the pears are poached to your liking, remove them from the liquid using a slotted spoon and let them cool slightly.

5. Serve the poached pears warm, drizzled with some of the poaching liquid, and garnished with a cinnamon stick if desired.

Nutritional Values (per serving):

- Calories: 160

- Protein: 1g

- Carbohydrates: 42g

- Dietary Fiber: 6g

Cooking Tip: Poaching pears in a fragrant mixture of apple juice, honey, or maple syrup, and warming spices like cinnamon creates a comforting and healthy dessert

Recipe 61: Mango and Chia Seed Pudding (no added sugars)

Prep Time: 10 minutes (plus chilling time) - Cooking Time: 0 minutes - Number of Servings: 4

Ingredients:

- 2 ripe mangoes peeled and diced.
- 1 cup unsweetened almond milk or any milk of your choice
- 1/2 cup chia seeds
- 1 tsp vanilla extract
- Fresh mango slices for garnish (optional)

Instructions:

1. In a blender, combine the diced mangoes and unsweetened almond milk.

2. Blend until smooth to create a mango puree.

3. In a mixing bowl, combine the mango puree, chia seeds, and vanilla extract.

4. Mix well to ensure the chia seeds are evenly distributed.

5. Cover the bowl and refrigerate for at least 2 hours or overnight to allow the chia seeds to absorb the liquid and create a pudding-like consistency.

6. Before serving, stir the mango and chia seed pudding to evenly distribute the chia seeds.

7. Optionally, garnish with fresh mango slices.

8. Serve the mango and chia seed pudding chilled.

Nutritional Values (per serving):

- Calories: 210

- Protein: 4g

- Carbohydrates: 31g

- Dietary Fiber: 10g

Cooking Tip: This no-added sugar mango and chia seed pudding is a wholesome and satisfying dessert or breakfast option. The chia seeds provide a delightful texture and add nutrition.

Recipe 62: Dark Chocolate Dipped Strawberries (minimal chocolate)

Prep Time: 15 minutes - Cooking Time: 0 minutes - Number of Servings: 4

Ingredients:

- 1 cup fresh strawberries washed and dried.
- 2 oz dark chocolate (70% cocoa or higher), chopped.
- 1/2 tsp coconut oil (optional for smoother chocolate)

Instructions:

1. In a microwave-safe bowl, combine the chopped dark chocolate and coconut oil (if using).

2. Microwave in 20-30-second intervals, stirring between each interval, until the chocolate is completely melted and smooth. Be careful not to overheat it.

3. Hold each strawberry by the stem and dip it into the melted chocolate, coating about two-thirds of the strawberry.

4. Allow any excess chocolate to drip back into the bowl.

5. Place the chocolate-dipped strawberries on a parchment paper-lined tray or plate.

6. Let the chocolate set at room temperature or, for quicker setting, place the tray in the refrigerator for about 15-20 minutes.

7. Once the chocolate is firm, serve the dark chocolate-dipped strawberries.

Nutritional Values (per serving):

- Calories: 70

- Protein: 1g

- Carbohydrates: 10g

- Dietary Fiber: 2g

Cooking Tip: Dark chocolate-dipped strawberries are a simple yet indulgent treat. Dark chocolate contains antioxidants and less sugar compared to milk chocolate, making it a better choice for a sweet treat.

Recipe 63: Vanilla and Berry Frozen Yogurt Bark (low-fat version)

Prep Time: 10 minutes (plus freezing time) - Cooking Time: 0 minutes - Number of Servings: 4

Ingredients:

- 2 cups low-fat plain Greek yogurt
- 2 tbsp honey or maple syrup (optional for added sweetness)
- 1 tsp vanilla extract
- 1 cup mixed berries (e.g., strawberries, blueberries, raspberries)
- 2 tbsp unsweetened shredded coconut (optional)
- Fresh mint leaves, for garnish (optional)

Instructions:

1. In a mixing bowl, combine the low-fat plain Greek yogurt, honey, maple syrup (if using), and vanilla extract. Mix well.

2. Line a baking sheet or tray with parchment paper.

3. Pour the yogurt mixture onto the parchment paper and spread it into an even layer, about 1/4-inch thick.

4. Sprinkle the mixed berries and unsweetened shredded coconut (if using) evenly over the yogurt.

5. Gently press the toppings into the yogurt.

6. Place the tray in the freezer and freeze for at least 2-3 hours or until the yogurt bark is firm.

7. Once frozen, break the bark into smaller pieces.

8. Optionally, garnish with fresh mint leaves.

9. Serve the vanilla and berry frozen yogurt bark straight from the freezer.

Nutritional Values (per serving, without honey/maple syrup or coconut):

- Calories: 100

- Protein: 7g

- Carbohydrates: 13g

- Dietary Fiber: 2g

Cooking Tip: This frozen yogurt bark is a light and satisfying dessert or snack, combining the creaminess of yogurt with the sweetness of berries. Customize it with your favorite fruits and toppings.

Chapter 11: Snack Recipes

Welcome to Chapter 11 of *"Pritikin Diet For Seniors: The Complete Guide to Weight Loss and Improved Health for Seniors."* In this chapter, we are thrilled to present a selection of nutritious and satisfying snack recipes that align perfectly with your health and longevity goals.

Our snack recipes have been carefully crafted to offer you a range of options that can keep you energized between meals without compromising your efforts to maintain a healthy body weight. We understand that snacking can be both enjoyable and beneficial for your well-being.

From crispy and savory delights to guilt indulgences, this chapter offers an array of choices to cater to different tastes and preferences. Each recipe has been thoughtfully designed using ingredients, ensuring that your snacks are not only nourishing but also deeply satisfying.

As you explore these snack recipes, you will realize that making decisions about your between-meal nibbles plays a role in embracing the Pritikin lifestyle. These snacks are specifically created not to curb cravings but to support your journey toward maintaining optimal body weight and improving overall health.

So join us on this journey through these snack recipes and discover how snacking can be an enjoyable and health-conscious part of your daily routine.

These recipes offer a variety of choices to fulfill your cravings and help you stay on track with your wellness objectives.

Chapter 11: Pritikin Snack Delights

64. Baked Kale Chips with a Sprinkle of Sea Salt

65. Fresh Vegetable Sticks with Hummus (low-fat version)

66. Spiced Roasted Chickpeas

67. Mixed Berry and Spinach Smoothie (no added sugars)

68. Cucumber Rounds Topped with Guacamole (low-fat version)

69. Oat and Date Energy Balls (no added sugars)

70. Edamame with a Sprinkle of Chili Flakes and Lemon Zest

These snack recipes are designed to provide quick energy boosts and curb hunger between meals while adhering to the Pritikin Diet's focus on whole foods and low fat.

Recipe 64: Baked Kale Chips with a Sprinkle of Sea Salt

Prep Time: 10 minutes - Cooking Time: 15 minutes - Number of Servings: 4

Ingredients:

- 1 bunch of fresh kale, stems removed and leaves torn into bite-sized pieces.
- 1 tbsp olive oil
- Sea salt, to taste

Instructions:

1. Preheat your oven to 350°F (175°C).

2. In a large bowl, toss the torn kale leaves with olive oil until they are lightly coated.

3. Spread the kale leaves in a single layer on a baking sheet.

4. Sprinkle a pinch of sea salt evenly over the kale.

5. Bake in the preheated oven for about 12-15 minutes or until the kale is crispy but not browned.

6. Remove from the oven and let the kale chips cool for a few minutes before serving.

Nutritional Values (per serving):

- Calories: 40

- Protein: 2g

- Carbohydrates: 6g

- Dietary Fiber: 1g

Cooking Tip: Baked kale chips are a crunchy and guilt-free snack. They're a great way to enjoy the health benefits of kale in a delicious form.

Recipe 65: Fresh Vegetable Sticks with Hummus (low-fat version)

Prep Time: 10 minutes - Cooking Time: 0 minutes - Number of Servings: 4

Ingredients:

- Assorted fresh vegetables (e.g., carrots, cucumber, bell peppers, celery) cut into sticks.
- 1 cup low-fat or fat-free hummus

Instructions:

1. Wash and prepare the assorted fresh vegetables by cutting them into sticks or spears.

2. Place the vegetable sticks on a serving platter.

3. Serve the fresh vegetable sticks with a side of low-fat or fat-free hummus for dipping.

Nutritional Values (per serving):

- Calories: 100

- Protein: 4g

- Carbohydrates: 18g

- Dietary Fiber: 6g

Cooking Tip: This snack provides a satisfying crunch and is a great way to enjoy a variety of fresh vegetables while dipping them in a tasty and nutritious low-fat hummus.

Recipe 66: Spiced Roasted Chickpeas

Prep Time: 5 minutes - Cooking Time: 25 minutes - Number of Servings: 4

Ingredients:

- 2 (15 oz.) cans of chickpeas, drained, rinsed, and patted dry
- 2 tbsp olive oil or avocado oil
- 1 tsp ground cumin
- 1/2 tsp paprika
- 1/2 tsp cayenne pepper (adjust to taste)
- Salt to taste

Nutritional Values (per serving):

- Calories: 230

- Protein: 10g

- Carbohydrates: 30g

- Dietary Fiber: 9g

Cooking Tip: Spicy roasted chickpeas make for a satisfying and crunchy snack. Adjust the level of cayenne pepper to your preferred spice level.

Instructions:

1. Preheat your oven to 400°F (200°C).

2. In a large bowl, combine the chickpeas, olive oil, ground cumin, paprika, and cayenne pepper. Toss until the chickpeas are evenly coated.

3. Spread the chickpeas on a baking sheet in a single layer.

4. Roast in the preheated oven for about 25 minutes, stirring or shaking the pan every 10 minutes, until the chickpeas are crispy and golden.

5. Remove from the oven and season with salt while still warm.

6. Allow the roasted chickpeas to cool completely before serving.

Recipe 67: Mixed Berry and Spinach Smoothie (no added sugars)

Prep Time: 5 minutes - Cooking Time: 0 minutes - Number of Servings: 2

Ingredients:

- 1 cup mixed berries (e.g., strawberries, blueberries, raspberries)
- 1 cup fresh spinach leaves
- 1 cup unsweetened almond milk or any milk of your choice
- 1/2 cup plain Greek yogurt (low-fat)
- 1/2 tsp vanilla extract
- Ice cubes (optional for thickness)
- Honey or maple syrup (optional for added sweetness)

Nutritional Values (per serving, without added sweetener):

- Calories: 90

- Protein: 6g

- Carbohydrates: 11g

- Dietary Fiber: 3g

Cooking Tip: This nutritious and no-added-sugar smoothie combines the goodness of mixed berries and spinach for a refreshing and energizing snack.

Instructions:

1. In a blender, combine the mixed berries, fresh spinach leaves, almond milk, plain Greek yogurt, and vanilla extract.

2. Optionally, add a few ice cubes to thicken the smoothie.

3. Blend until smooth and creamy. If desired, add honey or maple syrup for sweetness and blend again.

4. Pour the mixed berry and spinach smoothie into glasses and serve immediately.

Recipe 68: Cucumber Rounds Topped with Guacamole (low-fat version)

Prep Time: 10 minutes - Cooking Time: 0 minutes - Number of Servings: 4

Ingredients:

- 2 cucumbers, sliced into rounds.
- 1 ripe avocado peeled and mashed.
- 1 small tomato, diced.
- 1/4 cup diced red onion.
- 1/4 cup chopped fresh cilantro.
- Juice of 1 lime
- Salt and pepper to taste.
- Red pepper flakes (optional for added spice)

Nutritional Values (per serving):

- Calories: 80

- Protein: 2g

- Carbohydrates: 7g

- Dietary Fiber: 4g

Cooking Tip: These cucumber rounds topped with guacamole offer a refreshing and satisfying snack with a low-fat version of creamy guacamole.

Instructions:

1. In a bowl, combine the mashed avocado, diced tomato, diced red onion, chopped cilantro, and lime juice. Mix well.

2. Season the guacamole with salt, pepper, and red pepper flakes (if desired). Adjust to taste.

3. Slice the cucumbers into rounds.

4. Top each cucumber round with a spoonful of guacamole.

5. Optionally, garnish with additional chopped cilantro or red pepper flakes.

6. Serve the cucumber rounds with guacamole immediately.

Recipe 69: Oat and Date Energy Balls (no added sugars)

Prep Time: 15 minutes - Cooking Time: 0 minutes - Number of Servings: 12

Ingredients:

- 1 cup old-fashioned oats
- 1 cup pitted dates
- 1/4 cup unsweetened almond butter or any nut butter of your choice
- 1/4 cup chopped nuts (e.g., almonds, walnuts)
- 1/4 cup unsweetened shredded coconut
- 1 tsp vanilla extract
- A pinch of salt

Instructions:

1. Place the pitted dates in a food processor and process until they form a sticky paste.

2. In a mixing bowl, combine the old-fashioned oats, date paste, almond butter, chopped nuts, unsweetened shredded coconut, vanilla extract, and a pinch of salt.

3. Mix until all the ingredients are well combined.

4. Take small portions of the mixture and roll them into bite-sized energy balls.

5. Place the energy balls on a tray lined with parchment paper.

6. Refrigerate for at least 30 minutes to allow the balls to firm up.

7. Once chilled, store the oat and date energy balls in an airtight container in the refrigerator.

Nutritional Values (per energy ball):

- Calories: 90

- Protein: 2g

- Carbohydrates: 11g

- Dietary Fiber: 2g

Cooking Tip: These oat and date energy balls are a healthy and portable snack that provides a quick energy boost without added sugars.

Recipe 70: Edamame with a Sprinkle of Chili Flakes and Lemon Zest

Prep Time: 5 minutes - Cooking Time: 5 minutes - Number of Servings: 4

Ingredients:

- 2 cups frozen edamame (shelled)
- Zest of 1 lemon
- Chili flakes, to taste
- Salt, to taste

Instructions:

1. Bring a pot of water to a boil and add a pinch of salt.

2. Add the frozen edamame to the boiling water and cook for about 5 minutes or until they are tender.

3. Drain the cooked edamame and transfer them to a serving bowl.

4. Sprinkle the lemon zest and chili flakes over the edamame.

5. Toss to coat the edamame evenly with the lemon zest and chili flakes.

6. Serve the edamame with a sprinkle of additional salt if desired.

Nutritional Values (per serving):

- Calories: 90

- Protein: 7g

- Carbohydrates: 7g

- Dietary Fiber: 4g

Cooking Tip: Edamame is a nutritious and protein-rich snack. Adding lemon zest and chili flakes gives it a zesty and slightly spicy kick.

Chapter 12: Drink Recipes

Welcome to Chapter 12 of "***Pritikin Diet For Seniors: The Complete Guide to Weight Loss and Improved Health for Seniors***." It's important to stay hydrated and choose beverages that support your health goals. In this chapter, we invite you to explore a collection of drink recipes that do that.

Our drink recipes are carefully designed to quench your thirst while promoting well-being and weight management. We firmly believe that what you drink can have an impact on your nutrition, which is why these recipes are thoughtfully crafted to align with this philosophy.

From invigorating smoothies and rich juices to creative alcoholic cocktails and herbal infusions, this chapter offers a wide range of beverage options suitable for different tastes and dietary preferences. Each recipe focuses on using ingredients that provide hydration, essential nutrients, and delightful flavors.

As you delve into these drink recipes, you'll realize that enjoying a crafted beverage can be both enjoyable and health-conscious as part of your routine. These recipes go beyond the drinks themselves; they're about nourishing your body in the way.

So, come along on this journey as we delve into drink recipes that elevate your hydration game while contributing to your longevity and well-being.

Discovering the wonders of drinks and making decisions about what we consume can be a delightful and crucial part of embracing the Pritikin lifestyle.

Chapter 12: Pritikin Drink Delights

71. Cucumber-Mint Hydration Cooler

72. Golden Turmeric and Ginger Tea

73. Spinach, Pineapple, and Flaxseed Smoothie

74. Refreshing Watermelon and Basil Aqua Fresca

75. Herbal Rosemary and Lemon Infusion

76. Mixed Berry and Green Tea Smoothie

77. Iced Chamomile and Lavender Relaxation Brew

These drink recipes are crafted to refresh, rejuvenate, and relax while staying in harmony with the Pritikin Diet principles, using natural ingredients without added sugars or artificial flavors.

Recipe 71: Cucumber-Mint Hydration Cooler

Prep Time: 10 minutes - Cooking Time: 0 minutes - Number of Servings: 2

Ingredients:

- 1 cucumber peeled and sliced.
- 8-10 fresh mint leaves
- 4 cups cold water
- Ice cubes
- Lemon slices for garnish (optional)

Instructions:

1. In a pitcher, combine the sliced cucumber and fresh mint leaves.

2. Pour cold water over the cucumber and mint.

3. Stir to combine.

4. Add ice cubes to the pitcher to chill the cooler.

5. Optionally, garnish with lemon slices.

6. Serve the cucumber-mint hydration cooler cold.

Nutritional Values (per serving):

- Calories: 10

- Protein: 0g

- Carbohydrates: 2g

- Dietary Fiber: 1g

Cooking Tip: This cucumber-mint hydration cooler is a refreshing and low-calorie beverage to keep you hydrated, especially on warm days.

Recipe 72: Golden Turmeric and Ginger Tea

Prep Time: 5 minutes - Cooking Time: 10 minutes - Number of Servings: 2

Ingredients:

- 2 cups water
- 1-inch piece of fresh ginger peeled and sliced
- 1 tsp ground turmeric
- 1 tsp honey (optional for sweetness)
- Juice of 1/2 lemon (optional)
- Black pepper (a pinch for better turmeric absorption)

Instructions:

1. In a saucepan, bring the water to a boil.

2. Add the sliced fresh ginger and ground turmeric to the boiling water.

3. Reduce the heat to low and let the mixture simmer for about 10 minutes.

4. Strain the tea into cups.

5. Optionally, add honey and a squeeze of lemon juice for sweetness and flavor.

6. Add a pinch of black pepper, as it can enhance the absorption of turmeric.

7. Stir well and serve the golden turmeric and ginger tea hot.

Nutritional Values (per serving, without honey or lemon):

- Calories: 5

- Protein: 0g

- Carbohydrates: 1g

- Dietary Fiber: 0g

Cooking Tip: Turmeric and ginger are known for their anti-inflammatory properties. This tea is soothing and provides a warm, comforting drink.

Recipe 73: Spinach, Pineapple, and Flaxseed Smoothie

Prep Time: 5 minutes - Cooking Time: 0 minutes - Number of Servings: 2

Ingredients:

- 2 cups fresh spinach leaves
- 1 cup fresh pineapple chunks
- 1 cup unsweetened almond milk or any milk of your choice
- 2 tbsp ground flaxseeds
- Honey or maple syrup (optional for added sweetness)
- Ice cubes (optional for thickness)

Instructions:

1. In a blender, combine the fresh spinach leaves, fresh pineapple chunks, almond milk, and ground flaxseeds.

2. Optionally, add honey or maple syrup for sweetness.

3. Add ice cubes if you prefer a thicker smoothie.

4. Blend until smooth and creamy.

5. Pour the spinach, pineapple, and flaxseed smoothie into glasses and serve immediately.

Nutritional Values (per serving, without added sweetener):

- Calories: 90

- Protein: 3g

- Carbohydrates: 15g

- Dietary Fiber: 4g

Cooking Tip: This green smoothie combines the freshness of spinach and the tropical sweetness of pineapple, making it a nutrient-packed drink.

Recipe 74: Refreshing Watermelon and Basil Aqua Fresca

Prep Time: 10 minutes - Cooking Time: 0 minutes - Number of Servings: 2

Ingredients:

- 2 cups fresh watermelon chunks (seeds removed)
- 8-10 fresh basil leaves
- 2 cups cold water
- Ice cubes
- Lime slices for garnish (optional)

Instructions:

1. In a blender, combine the fresh watermelon chunks and fresh basil leaves.

2. Blend until smooth.

3. Pour the watermelon and basil mixture into a pitcher.

4. Add cold water and stir to combine.

5. Add ice cubes to chill the aqua fresca.

6. Optionally, garnish with lime slices.

7. Serve the refreshing watermelon and basil aqua fresca cold.

Nutritional Values (per serving):

- Calories: 30

- Protein: 0g

- Carbohydrates: 7g

- Dietary Fiber: 1g

Cooking Tip: This aqua fresca is a hydrating and flavorful drink with the natural sweetness of watermelon and the aromatic touch of basil.

Recipe 75: Herbal Rosemary and Lemon Infusion

Prep Time: 5 minutes - Cooking Time: 5 minutes - Number of Servings: 2

Ingredients:

- 2 cups water
- 2 sprigs of fresh rosemary
- Zest of 1 lemon
- Lemon slices for garnish (optional)
- Honey or agave nectar (optional for added sweetness)

Instructions:

1. In a saucepan, bring the water to a boil.

2. Add the fresh rosemary sprigs and lemon zest to the boiling water.

3. Reduce the heat to low and let the mixture simmer for about 5 minutes.

4. Strain the infusion into cups.

5. Optionally, add honey or agave nectar for sweetness.

6. Garnish with lemon slices if desired.

7. Serve the herbal rosemary and lemon infusion hot.

Nutritional Values (per serving, without sweetener):

- Calories: 0

- Protein: 0g

- Carbohydrates: 0g

- Dietary Fiber: 0g

Cooking Tip: This herbal infusion combines the earthy aroma of rosemary with the refreshing citrus notes of lemon for a soothing and aromatic drink.

Recipe 76: Mixed Berry and Green Tea Smoothie

Prep Time: 5 minutes - Cooking Time: 0 minutes – Number of Servings: 2

Ingredients:

- 1 green tea bag
- 1 cup boiling water
- 1 cup mixed berries (e.g., strawberries, blueberries, raspberries)
- 1 banana
- 1 cup unsweetened almond milk or any milk of your choice
- Honey or maple syrup (optional for added sweetness)
- Ice cubes (optional for thickness)

Instructions:

1. Place the green tea bag in a cup and pour boiling water over it. Let it steep for a few minutes, then remove the tea bag and let the tea cool.

2. In a blender, combine the cooled green tea, mixed berries, banana, almond milk, and ice cubes (if desired).

3. Optionally, add honey or maple syrup for sweetness.

4. Blend until smooth and creamy.

5. Pour the mixed berry and green tea smoothie into glasses and serve immediately.

Nutritional Values (per serving, without added sweetener):

- Calories: 90

- Protein: 2g

- Carbohydrates: 22g

- Dietary Fiber: 4g

Cooking Tip: This smoothie combines the antioxidant benefits of green tea with the vibrant flavors of mixed berries and bananas for a refreshing drink.

Recipe 77: Iced Chamomile and Lavender Relaxation Brew

Prep Time: 5 minutes - Cooking Time: 5 minutes - Number of Servings: 2

Ingredients:

- 2 cups water
- 2 chamomile tea bags
- 1 tsp dried lavender buds (culinary-grade)
- Honey or agave nectar (optional for added sweetness)
- Lemon slices for garnish (optional)

Instructions:

1. In a saucepan, bring the water to a boil.

2. Add the chamomile tea bags and dried lavender buds to the boiling water.

3. Remove the saucepan from the heat and let the mixture steep for about 5 minutes.

4. Remove the tea bags and strain the infusion into cups.

5. Optionally, add honey or agave nectar for sweetness.

6. Garnish with lemon slices if desired.

7. Allow the Iced Chamomile and Lavender Relaxation Brew to cool completely, then refrigerate or serve over ice.

Nutritional Values (per serving, without sweetener):

- Calories: 0

- Protein: 0g

- Carbohydrates: 0g

- Dietary Fiber: 0g

Cooking Tip: This herbal infusion is perfect for winding down and relaxing, combining the soothing properties of chamomile and the gentle fragrance of lavender.

Chapter 13: Strategies for Long-Term Success

Developing Healthy Habits and Routines

When it comes to achieving long-term success, developing habits and routines is incredibly important. These habits and routines form the foundation for seniors to build a fulfilling and healthy lifestyle. By adopting behaviors and making choices, individuals can greatly improve their overall well-being and increase their chances of success in various areas of life.

One crucial step towards establishing habits and routines is prioritizing self-care. This means ensuring you get to sleep following a diet and practicing effective stress management techniques. Sufficient sleep is essential for both mental well-being as it allows the body to repair and recharge itself. Seniors should aim for seven to eight hours of quality sleep each night while also establishing a bedtime routine that promotes sleep quality.

Another important aspect of self-care is maintaining a diet that focuses on foods like fruits, vegetables, whole grains, lean proteins, and healthy fats. Moderation is key here, so seniors should be mindful of portion sizes to avoid overeating. Additionally, staying hydrated throughout the day by drinking plenty of water is vital.

Overcoming Emotional Eating in Seniors

Eating is an issue, especially among older adults, and it can hinder their ability to maintain a healthy lifestyle in the long run. Emotional eating refers to the habit of turning to food as a way to deal with emotions or the stress of satisfying physical hunger. To overcome eating, seniors need to develop strategies for coping that don't involve food.

One effective approach is identifying the emotions that trigger the urge to eat. By recognizing and acknowledging these emotions, seniors can address the root causes. Discover ways of managing them. Engaging in activities like journaling, confiding in a trusted friend or therapist, or practicing relaxation techniques such as breathing or meditation can help shift their focus from food.

Furthermore, creating a positive environment is crucial for minimizing triggers that lead to eating. This involves surrounding oneself with a support system, participating in activities, and avoiding situations that induce excessive stress or negative emotions. By adopting coping mechanisms and fostering an environment, seniors can successfully conquer emotional eating and make lasting progress towards a healthier lifestyle.

Staying Active and Incorporating Exercise

Incorporating activity into daily routines plays an essential role in achieving long-term success. Regular physical exercise offers benefits for both the body and mind. It can improve health, increase strength and flexibility, enhance mood, and reduce the risk of illnesses.

If you're looking to stay active, it's important to have a rounded exercise routine that includes various types of activities. Aerobic exercises like walking, swimming, cycling, or dancing are options as they can be adapted to fitness levels.

Strength training exercises such as lifting weights or using resistance bands help maintain muscle mass and bone density, which in turn reduces the risk of falls and fractures. Additionally, flexibility exercises like stretching or practicing yoga improve mobility and overall flexibility.

Before starting any exercise program, especially if you have existing medical conditions, it is crucial to consult with healthcare professionals who can provide guidance based on your individual capabilities and health considerations. They will help you choose exercises that align with your needs.

To ensure long-term success and motivation in your fitness journey, it's important to track your progress. This allows you to monitor your achievements and identify areas where you can improve. By increasing the duration and intensity of activity while starting slowly at first, you'll prevent injuries and maintain consistency in the long run.

Seniors have a range of methods at their disposal to keep tabs on their progress. They can maintain a diary documenting their food intake and exercise, rely on smartphone apps, or make use of fitness devices. These tools play a role in keeping individuals accountable and motivated by offering insights into their habits and behaviors.

Furthermore, staying necessitates the establishment of goals and celebrating small victories along the way. Seniors should set both term and long-term objectives that align with their well-being goals. Breaking down goals into attainable milestones allows for a consistent sense of progress and boosts motivation. Celebrating these milestones, whether through treating oneself to a reward or sharing achievements with loved ones, reinforces behaviors and encourages ongoing progress.

To sum up, fostering habits and routines is essential for long-term success. By prioritizing self-care, overcoming eating tendencies, staying physically active, and tracking progress diligently, seniors can pave the way toward a more fulfilling lifestyle. Implementing these strategies consistently establishes a foundation for seniors to thrive in aspects of life while working towards achieving their long-term objectives.

Chapter 14: Addressing Common Concerns and Challenges

Dealing with Food Cravings and Temptations

Maintaining a healthy diet can be challenging, especially when faced with food cravings and temptations. Whether it's the desire for sugary treats or indulging in high-calorie meals, understanding how to handle these cravings is crucial for successful long-term dietary management.

Identify the root cause: It's essential to recognize the underlying reasons behind your food cravings. Are you truly hungry, or are you seeking comfort or distraction? Identifying triggers can help you find healthier alternatives or strategies to address the cravings effectively.

Stock up on healthy alternatives: Keep your pantry and refrigerator filled with nutritious snacks to help combat cravings. Fresh fruits, cut vegetables, whole-grain crackers, and low-fat yogurt are excellent options to satisfy hunger without compromising your health goals.

Practice portion control: It's okay to occasionally indulge in your favorite foods, but be mindful of portion sizes. Instead of completely denying yourself, enjoy smaller portions to satisfy your cravings without going overboard.

Distract yourself: Engage in activities that divert your attention away from food cravings. Go for a walk, read a book, listen to music, or call a friend. By focusing on something else, you can overcome the momentary craving and regain control.

Handling Social Situations and Dining Out

Social situations and dining out can present unique challenges when trying to adhere to a specific dietary plan. However, with proper planning and strategies, it is possible to navigate these situations without compromising your health goals.

Communicate your needs: Inform your friends, family, or hosts about your dietary preferences or restrictions in advance. This allows them to accommodate your needs and ensures there are suitable options available for you.

Research the menu: Before dining out, review the menu online to identify healthier choices. Look for dishes that are grilled, baked, or steamed, and ask for dressings or sauces on the side. Many establishments now offer lighter or modified versions of popular dishes.

Be mindful of portion sizes: Restaurants often serve large portions, which can lead to overeating. Consider sharing a dish with a friend or ask for a take-out container to save leftovers for another meal.

Focus on socializing: Instead of making the meal the primary focus of the gathering, shift your attention towards enjoying the company of others. Engage in conversation and participate in activities that don't revolve solely around food.

Managing Stress and Emotional Well-being

Stress and emotions can have a significant impact on our eating habits. Many individuals turn to food as a means of comfort or stress relief, which can lead to unhealthy eating patterns. Learning to manage stress and emotional well-being is vital for maintaining a healthy lifestyle.

Find alternative coping mechanisms: Instead of reaching for food during times of stress or emotional distress, explore other strategies that provide relief. Engaging in physical activity, practicing relaxation techniques like meditation or deep breathing, or pursuing hobbies can help distract from emotional triggers.

Seek support: Reach out to friends, family, or a support group to share your feelings and experiences. Surrounding yourself with a strong support system can offer encouragement and provide healthier outlets for emotional support.

Practice self-care: Prioritize self-care activities that help reduce stress and promote emotional well-being. This can include getting enough sleep, practicing mindfulness, engaging in regular physical activity, and setting aside time for activities you enjoy.

Tips for Dining in Assisted Living Facilities or Nursing Homes

For those residing in assisted living facilities or nursing homes, maintaining a nutritious diet can be a challenge. However, with some knowledge and advocacy, it is possible to make healthier choices and enjoy satisfying meals.

Communicate with staff and caregivers: Speak openly about your dietary needs, preferences, and any allergies or restrictions you may have. This will help ensure they are aware of your requirements and can provide suitable meal options.

Explore the menu options: Most facilities offer a variety of meal choices. Take the time to review the menu and select options that align with your dietary goals and restrictions. Don't hesitate to ask for modifications or substitutions if needed.

Engage in meal planning: If allowed, participate in meal planning or offer suggestions to the facility's staff. By providing input, you can help shape the menu to accommodate your preferences and dietary needs within reason.

Seek support from fellow residents: Connect with other residents who share similar dietary concerns or goals. Sharing experiences and tips can offer new ideas and build a sense of camaraderie, making the dining experience more enjoyable.

In conclusion, addressing common concerns and challenges related to diet and nutrition is crucial for maintaining a healthy lifestyle. By effectively dealing with food cravings and temptations, handling social situations and dining out, managing stress and emotional well-being, and utilizing tips for dining in assisted living facilities or nursing homes, individuals can successfully navigate these obstacles.

Remember, healthy eating is a lifelong journey. With determination, planning, and support, it is possible to achieve and maintain your desired dietary goals.

Chapter 15: Maintaining a Healthy Body Weight as You Age

As we get older, it becomes increasingly important to maintain a weight for our well-being and longevity. Keeping a weight not only improves our quality of life but also lowers the risk of developing chronic diseases like heart disease, diabetes, and certain types of cancer. In this chapter, we'll delve into why maintaining weight is crucial as we age, the significance of checkups and medical monitoring adapting the Pritikin Diet to specific health conditions, and lifestyle tips for enhancing our overall well-being.

The Significance of Regular Check-ups and Medical Monitoring

Regular checkups and medical monitoring are essential in keeping weight as we age. By monitoring our health and body weight, healthcare professionals can identify any concerns or underlying conditions that might hinder our efforts to manage our weight effectively. Regular checkups also give us an opportunity to evaluate how well our diet and lifestyle choices are working for us and make any adjustments. With the guidance of healthcare experts, we can promptly address any health issues that arise and establish a plan to maintain body weight.

Adapting the Pritikin Diet for Different Health Conditions

The Pritikin Diet is well known for its emphasis on foods and is a great way to achieve and maintain a healthy weight. However, it's important to customize this diet to meet health needs that may arise as we get older. For example, individuals with diabetes might need to pay attention to their carbohydrate intake and spread it out evenly throughout the day.

Those with heart disease could benefit from reducing sodium consumption and focusing on heart fats. Adapting the Pritikin Diet based on health conditions ensures that we can continue enjoying its benefits while addressing requirements.

Tips for Improving Overall Well-being through Lifestyle Choices

From following a diet, various lifestyle factors play a role in maintaining a healthy weight as we age. Incorporating activity into our daily routine is crucial because it not only helps manage weight but also enhances cardiovascular health, strengthens muscles and bones, and improves overall well-being. Activities like walking, swimming, or practicing yoga can be both enjoyable and beneficial.

Additionally, managing stress levels effectively and getting sleep are vital for maintaining weight.

Chronic stress has the potential to cause weight gain and make it harder to lose weight. That's why it's beneficial to practice stress-reducing techniques, like meditation or engaging in hobbies. It's also important to make sure we get to sleep each night as it supports our body's natural processes, including weight regulation.

Additionally, fostering an environment becomes increasingly important as we age for our overall health and well-being. Participating in activities, staying connected with friends and family, and seeking support from like-minded individuals can have a positive impact on our mental and emotional health. This, in turn, plays a role in maintaining body weight.

In summary, maintaining body weight as we age is crucial for living a healthy life. Check-ups and medical monitoring help identify any health conditions that may affect our efforts to manage our weight. Adapting the Pritikin Diet according to health conditions allows us to continue enjoying its benefits.

Additionally, incorporating activity into our lives, managing stress effectively, prioritizing quality sleep, and nurturing a supportive social environment are all vital lifestyle factors for maintaining a healthy body weight. By focusing on these aspects, we can improve our being and promote longevity.

Chapter 16: Conclusion

Recapping the Key Points

Throughout this book, we've delved into a range of topics. Shared valuable insights to help seniors navigate the challenges and opportunities that come with aging. As we reach the end of this journey, let us review the points and takeaways that can empower and inspire seniors to make the most out of their years.

First and foremost, we've emphasized the significance of maintaining a mindset and embracing an approach to aging. While it is natural to experience mental and emotional changes as we grow older, it's crucial to remember that age is a number. By cultivating positivity, setting goals, and prioritizing our well-being, we can continue leading fulfilling lives of vibrancy.

We've also discussed the importance of staying socially connected and engaged. Loneliness and isolation can have effects on our well-being. Therefore, seeking companionship and participating in activities that bring us joy are essential. Whether it entails joining clubs or organizations, volunteering our time, or taking part in community events—sustaining social connections enriches our lives while giving us a sense of purpose.

Furthermore, we've explored how taking care of our health plays a role...Regular physical activity, a balanced diet, and taking healthcare measures are all important for maintaining our vitality and independence. It's never too late to adopt habits or make changes to our lifestyle that can improve our overall well-being.

For all the seniors reading this book, we want to offer words of encouragement and inspiration. Remember that you have a wealth of life experiences and wisdom that can greatly benefit others. Embrace your journey. Share your knowledge with those around you. Consider becoming a mentor, getting involved in community volunteering, or even exploring career opportunities or business ventures. Your age should never hinder you from pursuing your passions and dreams.

Prioritizing self-care is also crucial: engage in activities that bring you joy. Whether it's spending time in nature pursuing hobbies or discovering interests, be sure to set aside time for yourself. By nurturing your well-being, you can continue to thrive and serve as an inspiration to others.

Here are some helpful resources. Suggested readings to assist you as you navigate the aspects of aging:

1. "Healthy Aging: A Lifelong Guide to Your Physical and Spiritual Well-Being" by Andrew Weil, M.D. This comprehensive book provides insights into maintaining your health as you age, covering mental and spiritual well-being.

2. "The Gift of Years: Growing Gracefully" by Joan Chittister. This profound exploration delves into both the joys and challenges of aging, offering guidance on finding meaning and purpose during stages of life.

3. "Aging Well: Surprising Guideposts to a Happier Life from the Landmark Harvard Study of Adult Development" by George E. Vaillant. Drawing upon a study on aging, this book offers advice and tips for living a fulfilling life as you grow older.

4. AARP (www.aarp.org). The website for the American Association of Retired Persons (AARP) provides a wealth of resources, information, and opportunities specifically tailored for seniors.

5. Local senior centers and community organizations are worth exploring in your area as they offer resources such as connections, educational programs, support groups, and services geared towards meeting the needs of older individuals.

These resources can be invaluable in your journey toward understanding aging and making the most out of this stage in life.

Remember, it's important to have knowledge and stay updated on the research, trends, and resources. This will help you make decisions and improve your well-being as you grow older.

To sum up, don't view aging as something to fear or endure. Instead, see it as a chance to embrace and celebrate life. By maintaining a mindset, staying socially active, taking care of our health, and pursuing our passions, we can lead a fulfilling and purposeful life at any age. As you enter the phase of your journey, remember that you're never alone. Opportunities are waiting for you to explore. Approach them with enthusiasm. May your senior years be filled with happiness, personal growth, and fulfillment.

Chapter 17: 14-day Meal Plan

Introducing the 14-Day Pritikin Meal Plan

When it comes to improving our health and vitality, the choices we make at mealtime play a role. The comprehensive cookbook that outlines the Pritikin Diet encourages us to embrace a lifestyle centered around nourishing and wholesome foods. This 14-day meal plan is more than a compilation of recipes: it serves as a guide to achieving wellness and longevity.

Adhering to a structured meal plan like the one featured in this book holds importance for various reasons deeply rooted in the core principles of the Pritikin Diet:

1. Attaining Optimum Health: The primary goal of the Pritikin Diet is to support health and well-being. By following this meal plan, you'll provide your body with nutrients for proper functioning. These nutrients include vitamins, minerals, fiber, and antioxidants—known to reduce the risk of ailments like heart disease, diabetes, and hypertension.

2. Sustainable Weight Management: Effective weight management goes beyond diets; it involves making lasting changes in our eating habits. The Pritikin Diet is known for its ability to promote weight loss and help individuals maintain it in the run.

3. Better Blood Sugar Management: The meal plan of the Pritikin Diet incorporates grains, legumes, and fruits, which are great options for stabilizing blood sugar levels. Following this plan consistently can help prevent spikes and drops in blood sugar, which is particularly beneficial for those with diabetes or at risk of developing it.

4. Heart Health Support: The emphasis on consuming sodium and saturated fat foods in the Pritikin Diet is beneficial for cardiovascular well-being. By sticking to this meal plan, you can lower your cholesterol levels, reduce blood pressure, and decrease your chances of heart disease.

5. Enhanced. Vitality: Nourishing your body with foods provides it with the energy required to thrive. When you consistently follow the Pritikin Diet, you'll experience increased energy levels, improved focus, and an overall sense of well-being.

6. Longevity Benefits: The goal of the Pritikin Diet isn't longevity but a better quality of life. By adhering to this meal plan, you provide your body with opportunities for an active and fulfilling life.

To successfully follow this 14-day meal plan, it's important to keep in mind the significance of preparation, mindful eating, and staying motivated. Make sure to plan your meals in advance, create grocery lists, and consider batch cooking for convenience. Practice portion.

Be mindful while eating to appreciate the flavors and textures of your meals. Always remember the impact that consistently following the Pritikin Diet can have on your health and overall quality of life.

Every day, as you enjoy the nutritious recipes provided, you'll be taking a step closer to becoming the healthier version of yourself that you've always wanted to be. Keep in mind that a meal plan is a tool to achieve your health goals. With dedication and commitment, you can experience the transformative benefits of the Pritikin Diet. So, let us embark on this 14-day journey towards health, one nourishing meal at a time.

Day 1:

Breakfast: Recipe 1 - Quinoa and Mixed Berry Bowl with Citrus Zest

Lunch: Recipe 15 - Mixed Bean Salad with Fresh Cilantro and Lime Dressing

Main Course: Recipe 29 - Grilled Lemon-Herb Tilapia with Asparagus Spears

Side: Recipe 43 - Garlic Steamed Green Beans with Toasted Almonds

Dessert: Recipe 57 - Chilled Melon Balls with Fresh Mint and Lime Zest

Drink: Recipe 71 - Cucumber-Mint Hydration Cooler

Day 2:

Breakfast: Recipe 7 - Steel-cut oats with Cinnamon, Apple, and Walnuts

Lunch: Recipe 26 - Stuffed Bell Peppers with Brown Rice and Black Beans

Main Course: Recipe 35 - Barley Risotto with Mushrooms and Green Peas

Side: Recipe 44 - Roasted Root Vegetables with Fresh Rosemary

Dessert: Recipe 58 - Baked Apples Stuffed with Oats and Raisins

Drink: Recipe 72 - Golden Turmeric and Ginger Tea

Day 3:

Breakfast: Recipe 14 - Pineapple and Mango Overnight Oats with Almond Slivers

Lunch: Recipe 20 - Spicy Chickpea and Kale Stew

Main Course: Recipe 40 - Vegetable Paella with Saffron and Artichokes

Side: Recipe 50 - Broccoli and Cauliflower Florets with Tahini Drizzle

Dessert: Recipe 59 - Berry and Kiwi Fruit Salad with a Lemon-Honey Drizzle

Drink: Recipe 73 - Spinach, Pineapple, and Flaxseed Smoothie

Day 4:

Breakfast: Recipe 11 - Zucchini and Corn Breakfast Burritos (whole grain tortillas)

Lunch: Recipe 23 - Roasted Beet and Orange Salad on a Bed of Arugula

Main Course: Recipe 37 - Steamed Cod with Ginger and Scallion Sauce

Side: Recipe 53 - Sweet Corn and Edamame Succotash

Dessert: Recipe 60 - Cinnamon-Spiced Poached Pears

Drink: Recipe 74 - Refreshing Watermelon and Basil Aqua Fresca

Day 5:

Breakfast: Recipe 3 - Spinach and Mushroom Breakfast Scramble (no oil)

Lunch: Recipe 24 - Zucchini Noodles Tossed in Fresh Tomato and Basil Sauce

Main Course: Recipe 33 - Grilled Eggplant and Tomato Stacks with Basil Drizzle

Side: Recipe 46 - Sautéed Kale with Golden Raisins and Pine Nuts (minimal oil)

Dessert: Recipe 61 - Mango and Chia Seed Pudding (no added sugars)

Drink: Recipe 75 - Herbal Rosemary and Lemon Infusion

Day 6:

Breakfast: Recipe 9 - Fresh Fruit Salad with a Splash of Orange Juice

Lunch: Recipe 16 - Grilled Veggie Wraps in Whole Wheat Tortillas with Hummus Spread

Main Course: Recipe 31 - Chickpea and Vegetable Curry over Brown Rice

Side: Recipe 47 - Grilled Asparagus Spears with Lemon Zest

Dessert: Recipe 62 - Dark Chocolate Dipped Strawberries (minimal chocolate)

Drink: Recipe 76 - Mixed Berry and Green Tea Smoothie

Day 7:

Breakfast: Recipe 5 - Whole Grain Toast with Smashed Avocado and Cherry Tomatoes

Lunch: Recipe 28 - Fresh Spring Rolls with Vegetables and a Tangy Tamarind Dipping Sauce

Main Course: Recipe 34 - Lentil and Vegetable Shepherd's Pie Topped with Cauliflower Mash

Side: Recipe 52 - Brussel Sprouts with Balsamic Reduction and Cranberries

Dessert: Recipe 63 - Vanilla and Berry Frozen Yogurt Bark (low-fat version)

Drink: Recipe 77 - Iced Chamomile and Lavender Relaxation Brew

Day 8:

Breakfast: Recipe 12 - Banana and Blueberry Smoothie with Chia Seeds (no added sugars)

Lunch: Recipe 21 - Cold Cucumber and Dill Soup with a Touch of Garlic

Main Course: Recipe 39 - Seared Tofu Steaks with Broccoli and Peanut Sauce (low-fat version)

Side: Recipe 54 - Baked Spinach and Artichoke Dip (low-fat version)

Dessert: Recipe 58 - Baked Apples Stuffed with Oats and Raisins

Drink: Recipe 72 - Golden Turmeric and Ginger Tea

Day 9:

Breakfast: Recipe 8 - Broccoli and Red Pepper Egg White Omelette

Lunch: Recipe 25 - Eggplant Roll-Ups with Spinach and Ricotta (low-fat) Filling

Main Course: Recipe 41 - Lemon-Pepper Roasted Brussels Sprouts and Tempeh Bowl

Side: Recipe 45 - Cilantro-Lime Brown Rice Pilaf

Dessert: Recipe 59 - Berry and Kiwi Fruit Salad with a Lemon-Honey Drizzle

Drink: Recipe 73 - Spinach, Pineapple, and Flaxseed Smoothie

Day 10:

Breakfast: Recipe 10 - Rye Pancakes Topped with Stewed Berries (no added sugars)

Lunch: Recipe 17 - Lentil Soup with Spinach and Diced Tomatoes

Main Course: Recipe 42 - Moroccan Vegetable and Chickpea Tagine

Side: Recipe 51 - Warm Beet Salad with Orange Segments

Dessert: Recipe 57 - Chilled Melon Balls with Fresh Mint and Lime Zest

Drink: Recipe 75 - Herbal Rosemary and Lemon Infusion

Day 11:

Breakfast: Recipe 4 - Chilled Melon Soup with Fresh Mint

Lunch: Recipe 19 - Grilled Portobello Mushrooms Stuffed with Spinach and Roasted Peppers

Main Course: Recipe 36 - Black Bean and Corn Stuffed Poblano Peppers

Side: Recipe 56 - Roasted Red Pepper and Walnut Spread (low-fat version)

Dessert: Recipe 60 - Cinnamon-Spiced Poached Pears

Drink: Recipe 74 - Refreshing Watermelon and Basil Aqua Fresca

Day 12:

Breakfast: Recipe 2 - Flaxseed and Oat Bran Muffins with Fresh Berries

Lunch: Recipe 15 - Mixed Bean Salad with Fresh Cilantro and Lime Dressing

Main Course: Recipe 30 - Stuffed Acorn Squash with Quinoa, Cranberries, and Spinach

Side: Recipe 55 - Quinoa and Black Bean Salad with Mango and Avocado

Dessert: Recipe 62 - Dark Chocolate Dipped Strawberries (minimal chocolate)

Drink: Recipe 71 - Cucumber-Mint Hydration Cooler

Day 13:

Breakfast: Recipe 7 - Steel-cut oats with Cinnamon, Apple, and Walnuts

Lunch: Recipe 22 - Whole Grain Pasta Salad with Mixed Vegetables and Lemon Vinaigrette

Main Course: Recipe 35 - Barley Risotto with Mushrooms and Green Peas

Side: Recipe 48 - Mashed Butternut Squash with a Hint of Nutmeg

Dessert: Recipe 58 - Baked Apples Stuffed with Oats and Raisins

Drink: Recipe 76 - Mixed Berry and Green Tea Smoothie

Day 14:

Breakfast: Recipe 14 - Pineapple and Mango Overnight Oats with Almond Slivers

Lunch: Recipe 26 - Stuffed Bell Peppers with Brown Rice and Black Beans

Main Course: Recipe 40 - Vegetable Paella with Saffron and Artichokes

Side: Recipe 50 - Broccoli and Cauliflower Florets with Tahini Drizzle

Dessert: Recipe 63 - Vanilla and Berry Frozen Yogurt Bark (low-fat version)

Drink: Recipe 77 - Iced Chamomile and Lavender Relaxation Brew

Appendix:

In this appendix, we present an extensive food list that outlines the foods you are encouraged to include in your diet while following the Pritikin program. Additionally, we have included a glossary to help you understand concepts and terms related to weight management. The principles discussed throughout this book.

Comprehensive List of Recommended Foods on the Pritikin Diet:

Fruits: Enjoy a wide variety of fresh fruits like apples, oranges, berries, melons, and more. It is advisable to limit dried fruits and fruit juices due to their sugar content.

Vegetables: Include a range of starchy vegetables in your meals, such as broccoli, kale, spinach, peppers, carrots, and more. Make sure to incorporate colors for nutritional benefits.

Whole Grains: Opt for grains like rice, quinoa, oats, barley, whole wheat bread, and whole grain pasta. These choices provide you with fiber, essential nutrients, and sustained energy levels.

Legumes: legumes such as beans (kidney beans or black beans), lentils, or chickpeas into your diet as they're excellent sources of protein, fiber, and vital minerals. These legumes also contribute towards satiety while helping maintain blood sugar levels.

Lean Sources of Protein: Opt for skinless poultry fish like salmon and trout, tofu, tempeh, and non-fat dairy products such as yogurt and cottage cheese. It's advisable to limit your intake of meat and choose cuts occasionally.

Incorporate Healthy Fats: Include foods that are rich in fats like avocados, nuts (such as almonds, walnuts, and cashews), and seeds (like flaxseeds and chia seeds). These fats are beneficial for heart health. Help you feel satisfied.

Enhance Flavor with Herbs and Spices: Add a variety of herbs and spices to your meals for taste. Basil oregano, turmeric, and cinnamon paprika are choices. This allows you to enjoy meals without relying on salt or unhealthy condiments.

Foods Not Recommended on the Pritikin Diet:

Avoid Processed Foods: Stay from processed foods like fast food, packaged snacks, and sugary beverages, as they tend to be high in added sugars, unhealthy fats, and artificial ingredients.

Minimize Refined Grains: Reduce consumption of rice, white bread, refined cereals, and pastries, as these lack nutrients and can cause blood sugar spikes.

Say No to Added Sugars: Steer clear of foods and drinks that contain added sugars, such as soda, candy pastries, and sweetened cereals. Choose sweetness from fruits instead.

Limit your consumption of foods in saturated fats: Stay away from fatty cuts of meat, dairy products, and butter. It's best to avoid trans fats, which are often found in processed snacks and fried foods, as they can have effects on heart health.

Watch High Sodium Foods: Reduce the number of high-sodium foods you eat, such as processed meats, canned soups, and salted snacks. Instead, enhance the flavor of your food by using herbs, spices, and natural seasonings.

Glossary:

Weight Management: The process of adopting habits and making lifestyle changes to achieve and maintain body weight. This involves following a diet, engaging in physical activity, and modifying behavior.

Pritikin Diet: A nutrition plan developed by Nathan Pritikin that focuses on eating foods derived from plants. It emphasizes consuming fat and high-fiber foods with the goal of improving health, reducing the risk of chronic diseases, and promoting weight loss.

Fiber: A type of carbohydrate in plant-based foods that cannot be digested by the body. It aids in digestion and promotes a feeling of satiety or fullness after meals while helping regulate blood sugar and cholesterol levels.

Protein: Protein is a nutrient that plays a role in building and repairing tissues, supporting our immune system, and aiding in various metabolic processes. It is composed of acids. It can be obtained from both animal and plant sources.

Satiety: Satiety refers to the feeling of fullness and satisfaction we experience after a meal. Including foods that are rich in fiber, protein, and water content in our diet can enhance satiety levels, making it less likely for us to overeat.

Unsaturated fats: These fats are considered fats found in plant-based foods, as well as certain types of fish. These fats contribute to heart health, reduce inflammation, and support brain function.

To successfully adopt the Pritikin Diet and manage your weight effectively, it's important to familiarize yourself with the recommended and discouraged food options on this diet plan. By making choices based on these guidelines, you can embark on a journey towards a lifestyle. Remember that incorporating these changes is a step towards achieving your health goals while enhancing your overall well-being.

About The Author

Samantha Bax, an advocate of vegan, friendly, and renal-conscious cuisine, found her true calling in the heart of a bustling city. Her journey in a professional kitchen began in her grandmother's cozy home, where she first learned the value of wholesome and nutritious eating.

When Samantha was diagnosed with diabetes in her twenties, her life turned. This pivotal moment fueled her dedication to health and wellness, ultimately leading her to become a certified nutritionist. However, when a close family member was diagnosed with kidney disease, fate had a plan for Samantha. This significant event merged her two passions for food and well-being, inspiring her to create a niche catering to diabetic and renal diets.

Course Samantha encountered challenges along the way. Balancing health requirements with flavors proved to be complex. However, she refused to compromise taste for health's sake. To overcome this hurdle, Samantha embarked on a culinary adventure where she drew inspiration from kitchens across the Mediterranean region, spice markets in Asia, and farms throughout Central America.

In ***"Pritikin Diet For Seniors: The Complete Guide to Weight Loss and Improved Health for Seniors,"*** Samantha Bax masterfully combines her story with a collection of mouth-watering recipes. She firmly believes that while food is essential for survival, it should also be cherished as a celebration of life and well-being.

Outside of writing and culinary experimentation, Samantha finds joy in the art of photography. She captures the essence of both cityscapes and peaceful natural landscapes. Additionally, she leads workshops and seminars where she guides individuals in making food choices that don't compromise on taste.

To join our Newsletter and receive advance notification of new publications, subscribe to the Newsletter for FREE today at:

www.prosebooks.us/subscribe

Made in the USA
Columbia, SC
28 December 2023

29563185R10076